CARING FOR PEOPLE

Help at the frontline

Jenny Rogers

Open University Press
• Philadelphia

Open University Press
Celtic Court
22 Ballmoor
Buckingham
MK18 1XW

and
1900 Frost Road, Suite 101
Bristol, PA 19007, USA

First Published 1990
Reprinted 1993

British Library Cataloguing in Publication Data

Rogers, Jenny 1939–
    Caring for people.
    1. Great Britain. Care assistant services
    I. Title
    362.0425

    ISBN 0 335 09430 9
    ISBN 0 335 09429 5 (pbk)

Library of Congress Cataloging in Publication Data

Rogers, Jennifer
    Caring for people / by Jennifer Rogers.
        p.   cm.
    Includes bibliographical references and index.
    ISBN 0-335-09430-9 (hb). – ISBN 0-335-09429-5 (pb)
    1. Human services personnel – United States – Handbooks,
manuals, etc. 2. Caregivers – United States – Handbooks, manuals,
etc.
    I. Title.
    HV40.35.R64   1990
    361.3′2 – dc20   90-7640 CIP

Typeset by Colset Pte Ltd, Singapore
Printed in Great Britain by The Bath Press Ltd, Avon

Contents

Acknowledgements

Grateful acknowledgement is made to the following for permission to reproduce the illustrations:

The Open College for 'Positive body language', from *Managing Change*, 1989; British Coal for 'How to open the airway', 'The recovery position', 'Mouth-to-mouth breathing' and 'Chest compressions' from *British Coal Skill Scope*; and to Dorling Kindersley, The St. John Ambulance Association and Brigade, The St. Andrew's Ambulance Association and The British Red Cross Society for 'The abdominal thrust' from *The First Aid Manual*.

Introduction

This book assumes that you are a care support worker, fairly new to the job and interested in improving the understanding and skill you need to do your job well. You may perhaps work as a care assistant in a private or local authority residential home, as a home care assistant (home help), as an auxiliary in a hospital or as a trainee social worker.

A book cannot hope to cover all the many aspects of performing well in jobs which need such a wide range of skills. For that you will need to rely on training from your employer and the depth of knowledge that will come from experience. However, I have tried to highlight many of the topics in the work which both carers and their clients find important.

Care work is challenging because you are in the front line of care. The demands it will make on you are considerable:

- You are usually the person who has to deal first with clients who are frightened, upset, confused, angry and lonely. This takes sensitivity, courage and skill.
- You have to perform intimate tasks for people who would much rather do such things for themselves – if only they could. This takes cheerfulness, respect for other people's privacy and tact.
- You may have to deal with dying clients and bereaved relatives. This takes compassion and emotional strength.
- You have to decide how to exercise the considerable power you have to affect the lives of your clients. This takes self-knowledge, clear-sightedness and restraint.
- You need to be able both to talk and to listen skilfully. This takes exceptional ability to communicate.

- You have to cope with the stress of a job which is hard physically and demanding emotionally.

No wonder, then, that the job of providing care support has often been described as the most invisible professional work in our society: *invisible* perhaps because it is so often done by part-timers and by people who are chronically underpaid for what they do, *professional* because it demands skill of a high order.

But even if the work is badly paid, there is no doubt of its rewards in other ways, described here, first by an auxiliary in a convent hospital and then by a care officer for a voluntary society:

> I go home tired every day, but I *know* that my work is essential to the happiness and physical well-being of at least six people. I give a lot but, my word, so do they . . . I sat with a client last week who was dying and I held her hand and talked to her gently and she talked to me. I was with her and still holding her hand when she died. It was so peaceful – a beautiful death. It wrenches you when someone dies, but I know my work is vital and that I do it well.

> I wouldn't change my work for anything. OK, I'm only paid a pittance, but when you see something like I did today – a little girl of five with very severe cerebral palsy actually able to take a step unaided for the first time ever – I could have cried with joy. I have worked like stink for that child and today I got my reward!

This is work that touches the lives of the most vulnerable people in our society. How to cope with some of the problems and issues raised by such work is what the rest of this book is about.

1

The need for care

> I work in a home in a small country town. I still can't get over the fact that none of the twelve old ladies I look after ever has a visitor or even a letter from a friend. They seem to be abandoned people. I know *we* look after them, but after all, we're paid to do it, so it's not the same, is it?

> I have four regulars that I visit every day. If I didn't call, they literally wouldn't speak to anyone all day long. It's terrible for them to be so cut off from love and friendship.

Perhaps you, too, have shared the feelings expressed here by these two carers: feelings of indignation and pity that the people you help look after have apparently been abandoned by their families to the paid care of strangers. This chapter looks at some of the reasons why a job which barely existed 100 years ago is now often described as part of a 'growth industry' because so many people work in it. What is it that has changed so dramatically? Why is there a need for paid carers at all?

People are living longer

One of the main reasons for the growing need for carers, both paid and unpaid, is that the numbers of people needing care is increasing so quickly. You are likely to live longer than your parents, who in turn are likely to live longer than your grandparents, and your children are likely to live longer than you.

Why? Mainly because standards of living have risen steadily throughout the twentieth century. Higher standards of living normally mean better health. Take hygiene, for instance. When today's eighty-year-old was a child, it was perfectly acceptable to have a house with an outside non-flush lavatory. Even until the outbreak of the Second World War, many builders were still putting up houses without bathrooms. You do not have to be a public health expert to see that a lavatory which is just a hole in the ground, combined with a house where there is no constant hot water, is certain to make washing yourself a bit of a chore and infection more likely. Today, by contrast, many young couples aspire to own a two-bathroom house with central heating within a few years of setting up home together. Where clothes used to be washed once a week with enormous trouble in a 'copper' (a gas or coal-fired boiler), many of us now casually throw our clothes into an automatic washing machine after only one wearing.

Food storage, too, has changed, mostly for the better. Where once only the very rich were able to refrigerate food, now nine out of ten households have a refrigerator and six out of ten a freezer. How many people today would know what a 'meat safe' is? Yet as late as 1950, this simple wooden cupboard with a wire netting door was the most common kitchen defence against flies, although of course it offered no defence at all against the bacteria encouraged by not keeping food cool.

As food storage has changed, so has the food we eat. To the dismay of the government in the First World War, large numbers of recruits had to be rejected on medical grounds, the main reason being that they were suffering from severe malnutrition.

Even at the time of the Second World War there was still chronic and widespread poverty, which became embarrassingly obvious when thousands of city children were separated on safety grounds from their parents and sent as 'evacuees' to reluctant hosts in the country. One woman, now in her eighties, remembers how one such little group struck her own by no means rich family:

> These children had no possessions, not even suitcases. They had a few clothes in pillowcases, that was all. They were just skin and bone, all of them: so thin it was pathetic. As far as I could see they'd never ever had enough food. Their clothes stank because they were never washed and every last one of them had head lice. I can tell you that we loathed them; it was unfair, but we did, even though now I feel ashamed of how we treated them.

Today, such acute poverty is very uncommon, not least because technological change in equipment, fertilizers and farming methods has produced cheap food on a scale previously unimaginable: so much of it, indeed, that the grain and butter mountains and wine lakes of the European Community have become notorious. Even in this affluent society there are still many people who cannot spend freely on food – perhaps some of them are your clients – but serious malnutrition of the sort that was commonplace in the earlier years of the twentieth century is rare. Now, a bigger problem is the opposite to malnutrition – the over-nutrition which produces the 'diseases of affluence': heart disease, many cancers and digestive disorders, caused by eating too much fatty, highly refined food.

Technological development has also led to several changes that have improved standards of living and thus have tended to increase the length of time we live. One is the development of cheap and easily available contraception. As a result, women need no longer run the risks of repeated childbearing. This is probably the single most important element in improving the health of women in the twentieth century. Pregnancy and childbirth may be 'natural' events, but they are also risky. Fewer pregnancies normally means better health for women.

The reduction in typical family size has had other dramatic effects. When you only have one or two children to care for, your money goes further and you can care more effectively for the children you do have. Also, of course, motherhood is no longer a lifetime's job. Reduction in typical family size from five or six children to only one or two means that the childbearing years form a relatively short period of a woman's life. This power over our own bodies has been an important part of the new attitudes towards women, including of course, the attitudes women have about themselves. Along with the right to choose when you have a baby goes the right to choose not to have one at all, the right to choose to make your paid employment an important part of the rewards you expect from life and the right to expect to be able to compete with men if you want to. All this means that the army of unpaid carers who, in the past, lavishly and often uncomplainingly cared for the frailer members of their families can no longer be assumed to be there – or if they are, they cannot be assumed to be willing to take on such exacting roles.

One other significant technological-medical development of the twentieth century is the discovery of antibiotics in the 1940s. Before antibiotics, treatment for bacterial infections was not very effective. Otherwise fit and healthy people often died from infected wounds or from illnesses such as bronchitis and tuberculosis. If you look after elderly clients, they may be able to give you examples from their own families of people who died or were gravely ill in these circumstances. The experiences described by these elderly people are typical:

> My brother was in the Home Guard in the war. Someone dropped a tram rail they were taking up on to his feet. He had a terrible injury, developed gangrene and died. It makes me bitter even now to think that only a few years later, penicillin would probably have saved his life.

> I've always had a horror of colds and 'trivial' illnesses because in my childhood they so often turned into really dangerous things. As a child I was very ill with pneumonia. There was no antibiotic treatment and I nearly died.

It is highly likely that antibiotics will have had significant impact on the health of your clients and indeed your own. If you look after handicapped people, for instance, many of these clients are likely to owe their lives to this type of drug. Both babies with Down's syndrome and those born with spina bifida are at serious risk from infections that healthier people can shrug off easily. Antibiotic treatment means that many handicapped babies now survive into adult life, whereas fifty years ago they were lucky to survive infancy. Many such people will need institutional or other kinds of professional care for most of their lives. The existence of this and other modern treatments can also, of course, pose new dilemmas for relatives and carers, as this mother describes:

> What do we do about Robert's future? For a Down's person he is reasonably fit, quite intelligent and likely to live on to middle age. Since we were in our forties when we had him, he is pretty certain to outlive us. We are frantically trying to work out a way to set up a trust for him so that after our deaths he will be able to live in some pleasant, not-too-institutional home. Our plan is to find a suitable place, introduce him to it gradually so that he spends regular weekends there. It's an awful problem – preoccupies a lot of my thoughts at the moment.

It is not only the carers of the mentally handicapped who face such problems. Modern treatment may, for instance, prolong the lives of chronically ill elderly people to the point where, for months or even years, they are living a twilight existence only sustained by drugs and nursing. The auxiliary expresses common doubts about the morality of encouraging such a half-life:

> Many of our patients are very, very ill and don't know what day of the week it is a lot of the time. I do wonder, often, if it's right to prolong their lives like this. When their notes say things like 'not to be resuscitated' you do wonder what the point of all this aggressive therapy actually is.

Antibiotics have been, and continue to be, so important in modern medicine that it is hard to single out any one aspect over others, but perhaps it is worth mentioning one further way in which they have helped increase our longevity, and that is in controlling infections after surgery. You may, for instance, have elderly clients who have had hip replacements. This ingenious and common operation to treat the joint and bone damage caused by arthritis has been made possible by technological advances in the manufacture of the artificial joints themselves. Arthritis is not, in itself, life-threatening, but the existence of antibiotics means that if serious infection occurs after operations it can be controlled. The same is true of all surgery, whether it is for something minor like varicose veins, or for major operations to treat heart disease and cancer. Surgery of all sorts is thus much more likely to be successful because its complications can be far better controlled than in the days before antibiotics.

Public health has been better managed in the twentieth than in any previous century; for instance, campaigns to immunize against the major infectious diseases of childhood like measles, diphtheria and whooping cough have gone hand in hand with state commitment to providing clean water and efficient sewerage services.

In all these changes, and others like them, one change causes and feeds into another so that it is sometimes hard to see which is the cause and which the effect. For instance, some people have argued that mass immunization is not the cause of the decline in deaths from childhood illnesses, but is the result of increased prosperity which increases our natural immunity to disease. They point to illnesses like scarlet fever which were common in the earlier years of the twentieth century and which have now disappeared, even though there has been no immunization campaign against the disease. Here, it is possible both that the virus has changed and that our immunity to it has increased. Similarly, you could argue that the availability of contraception is only one part of the reason why people start having fewer children: standards of living usually have to increase first, so that, for instance, people start believing that the children they do have will survive infancy. In Third World countries where infant mortality is still high, people tend to opt for larger families in spite of major campaigns for free contraception. The reason is not only that children are seen as a vital part of the family economy, but also that parents still do not dare trust that all the children they have will actually live to grow up.

One other major change may prove to be of long-term significance in extending life span. This is the growing realization that prevention really *is* better than cure. The 1980s crazes for running, jogging, aerobics and muesli were not really the silly fads they might have appeared. All were based on solid medical evidence that how we live our lives – what we eat and drink and how much exercise we take – is just as important as anything the medical experts can do for us. Whereas, in previous generations, chronic ill-health was regarded as inevitable, the modern attitude is that your aim in life should be, as one health expert put it, 'to die healthy' – in other words to continue to lead an active and useful life into very old age. In the United States, where the message about stopping smoking, exercising seriously and eating prudently has been heeded for longer than in Britain, the rate of sudden deaths from heart disease has already noticeably fallen. If we follow the American trend, then the number of elderly people in Britain may increase even faster.

The balance of the population is changing

One reason why there are so many people now needing care is that the balance of the population is changing. More people are surviving into very old age at the same time as family size is falling. When so much of the population is middle-aged and elderly, it is inevitable that the responsibility for providing care will often have to fall outside the family. In this case, for instance, all the people involved are well into old age and have no adult children who can help:

> My sister married late and was widowed after only 15 years of marriage. She had been very babied by her husband and always said she needed someone to look after her. Unfor-

tunately, her husband was a spendthrift. When he died, she discovered for the first time that they were virtually penniless. She rented another, cheaper, flat and managed there for a while, then she had a serious stroke and it was obvious that she couldn't continue living alone. I suppose my wife and I could have taken her in, but this was not a realistic proposition. We married, each for the second time, in our sixties after we both became widowed. My wife had looked after her invalid first husband for ten years before he died and had also looked after his mother for five years before that. We were both seventy-five at the time of my sister's stroke. If my sister had had any capital we might have been able to buy something together, but of course she didn't and we couldn't. There was no option but to look for a place for her in a local authority home, even though it broke my heart to see her there.

Family and community life is changing

The fact that people are having fewer children than they did in the early years of the twentieth century has one immediate effect on the care of those who are too frail to look after themselves – there are fewer people who can even contemplate sharing the responsibility:

I dread my parents becoming confused or physically disabled as I am an only child. My mother looked after her mother in similar circumstances, but she was one of six and there was always a brother or sister handy to help out with shopping or to sit with her in the evenings.

Not so many years ago, people not only had more children, they also tended to live close to their adult children and grandchildren, sometimes even in the same street. A survey carried out in the 1950s by the sociologist, Peter Townsend, and reported in his classic book, *The Family Life of Old People*, revealed how common and important such contacts were:

Mrs Rilk, an infirm widow in her early sixties, lived alone. A married daughter living nearby regularly did her cleaning and gave her meals on Sundays. Her shopping was done by a thirteen-year-old grandson. 'He comes every morning before school.' As for washing, another grandson 'calls in when he's

on his milk round on Sunday and collects it. My daughter gets
it done on Monday and Charlie [the grandson] brings it back.'
Her grandchildren chopped firewood for her, exercised her dog
and took her to the cinema or to the bus-stop, her daughter
collected the pension. But Mrs Rilk prepared a meal for her
daughter and grandchildren six days of the week, often
entertained her relatives in the evenings, and once or twice
a week she took a meal to an old lady in the same block of flats.

Mrs Rilk was very typical of the elderly people in Bethnal Green,
London, whose lives were studied in the survey. Even where they
lived alone, very few of them were isolated. Those interviewed had
an average of thirteen relatives living within a mile and often saw
their adult children every day.

Today that pattern is breaking up. While there are still communities where you can see this 'extended family' pattern, it is becoming
increasingly rare. As children grow up, there may simply be no
suitable work for them: they have to move away. This has been
especially true in areas which were previously the centres of heavy
industry like mining and steel. Here is Thomas, now seventy-seven,
still living at home but supported by a home care assistant, talking
about why it is impossible for his two sons to look after him:

My boys grew up here in South Wales and I was determined
that they wouldn't have to go down the mines like I did and
like my father did, wrecking their health. In any case, the pits
are closing and everything else here depends on the pits, so
when that's finished there's nothing to keep them. But this
is my village – you wouldn't catch me moving to London or
Bristol even though they've both tried to persuade me to come
and live with them.

Even where adult children do still live reasonably near at hand,
there may be other forces at work which make the prospect of sharing
a home fraught for both sides, as in this case, described by the client's
home care assistant:

One of the ladies I look after still lives in the cottage where
she was born. She was the eldest of eight children and had to
work to support the younger ones from the age of fourteen.
She married a local chap and inherited the cottage from her
parents. It's pretty on the outside but horribly damp and cold

inside. She refuses to put carpet down – says lino's always been good enough for her. Yet her sideboard is crammed with pictures of her son, daughter and grandchildren: the son and daughter in graduation gear; the daughter meeting the Queen at some do or other; the granddaughters on ponies . . . I used to feel so sorry for her because there are her children leading very affluent lives and they don't seem to do much more than duty visits. But one day I happened to be there when her son rolled up, brand new car, accent you could cut with a knife, posh clothes, and I realized that the life he leads is just so totally different, thanks to the education she made sure he got, that it would be sentimental and silly to think that they could ever live together again.

The same sorts of forces are at work in this account, given this time by a middle-aged woman whose father-in-law has just moved into sheltered housing:

My father-in-law had to go into sheltered housing because he couldn't really go on in the awful old house he was in with his health being so dodgy and there was no way he could have lived with us. It sounds awful to put it so brutally, but the class differences would have made it ghastly. He spits and hawks and I've often caught him not using a handkerchief but expelling snot into a basin with his fingers. He eats different food at different times of day – these things sound trivial, but they're not when you have to confront them on a daily basis. I look at my husband and often wonder how on earth he came from this background to the job he now has as a writer and broadcaster.

You may know of many clients where this kind of story is common: elderly people whose own education was neglected for one reason or another, but who somehow saw to it that their children did better. The price paid has often been high: education and the nature of the work it has fitted their children to do have driven a wedge between them and their parents, making it virtually impossible for the adult children to contemplate looking after their parents.

Even where there is no difficulty of this type, family life itself is changing. The UK divorce rate is the highest in Europe and one of the highest in the world. Marriage breakdown, again, makes it harder for people to look after the physically or mentally frail members of their families. Divorce usually means less money and smaller houses, whereas the care of an elderly parent or a handicapped son or daughter may demand more money and a bigger house. Divorce and separation are themselves horribly painful experiences which leave everyone involved with little spare physical or emotional energy. This client's experience is representative of many others:

> We moved into sheltered housing because the only other possibility – pooling resources with our younger daughter – was never really on. She has just been through a traumatic separation from her husband where she's had to struggle to get anywhere to live because she has so little money. What is worse is that after 25 years of marriage she's having to get used to living alone and to seeing her former husband with a woman half her age. She's feeling very bruised and very rejected and we didn't feel it was fair to ask her to cope with us as well. My wife had a stroke last year and I have Parkinson's, so it wouldn't be much fun taking us on.

In the past, it was not only family members who helped look after the frailer people in the community: often the responsibility was shared by neighbours and friends. But this is only usually possible in a settled community where people have known each other well for many years – increasingly a rarity in a society where the average household now moves once every seven years. The reasons for such frequent moves are, again, the need to look for work, and the wish to develop a career through promotion.

Now that so many more people are house owners, a further reason for moving is the wish or need to respond to changing house prices. When house prices rise steeply, many people cash in their value in much the same way as people in other countries buy and sell shares. More frequent divorce, again, is responsible for a large number of house moves. All of this leads to the sort of community which makes it difficult for people to know their neighbours well, and unusual to have much of the informal, shared responsibility for the elderly or handicapped which was common in the past, and is remembered wistfully here by one home care assistant:

> I grew up in Bradford in a little terraced house in a street where everybody knew everybody. My sister lived in the same street

and had a disabled and mentally handicapped son, but it wasn't the problem it is today for families. Everybody knew him and helped keep an eye on him. If he wandered off, which he did sometimes, someone would bring him back and say 'Now come on Tommy, your mam's going to be worried about you' and give him a piece of cake to be going on with. He was just part of the scene. I often think about him now, as I'm now paid to help look after families with children like him – isn't it a shame that no one local will help?

There are other significant changes in patterns of family life. Many young people are not getting married at all: the fact that it is now perfectly acceptable to live together without having gone through a wedding ceremony is shown in statistics which reveal that one in four of all babies is now born to parents who are not married. A couple may be just as loyal to one another as if they were legally married, but it seems doubtful that they will feel the same intense sense of obligation to parents, aunts and uncles that probably distinguished the lives of their own families a generation or two ago.

The 'me first' generation

Looking back to an apparently golden age is always dangerous. Was there ever really a time, for instance, when people always respected their parents and when there wasn't a 'generation gap'? People's deepest feelings on these matters have probably always been rather similar. But certainly in the last quarter of the twentieth century there has been the chance not just to *think* 'me first' but to *act* on it. How far this has been encouraged by a political and economic climate which appears to put material success before family responsibility is difficult to judge.

Whatever your private views on the matter, it is wiser to avoid snap judgements. It will be difficult for you as a person on the outside of the family to understand all the complications of the relationships inside it which may lead a family to feel that they cannot provide care themselves:

> On the surface my parents appeared to be loving and respectable, but looking back on it, they gave me a perfectly awful childhood. They made it clear that I was a disappointment from

the start because I wasn't a boy, then I was a disappointment because I failed the eleven-plus, then I always answered back . . . I was often slapped and beaten, and, what was worse, my father was capable of sulking for weeks: he once went seven whole weeks without speaking to me. I was frequently punished by not being given food, then slapped again if hunger forced me to steal it and I got caught. Now they're old and my mother is frail. There's no way I could ever have them here: I just can't forgive them for what they did – my dad especially.

Perhaps deep-rooted family problems of a similar kind are at the back of the apparently inexplicable neglect of their parents by adult sons and daughters which so often irritates carers like this one:

One of the ladies at —— House, Mrs B, is very confused, but even so, it riles me that her daughter lives literally in the same street and hardly ever calls in, even when the matron sees her on the pavement and actually invites her in. Once, in a rare moment of clear-headedness, Mrs B suddenly said to me: 'My daughter doesn't visit me, you know'. I said: 'Oh yes, I know, isn't it a shame, why's that?' To my astonishment she replied, absolutely lucidly: 'She had a baby when she was only nineteen and I forced her to give it up for adoption. That seemed the right thing to do at the time, but she blames me for the whole thing.' I don't *think* this was fantasy – it sounded like the truth. If so, it explains a lot.

The growth of state care

If you look after elderly clients, they will certainly remember the shame and horror of 'the workhouse'. For many centuries until comparatively recently, this was the only place in which the frail and destitute could be helped. To be reduced to admission to a workhouse was to admit total defeat: a life where men and women had to live separately, where food was meagre and where self-esteem was deliberately blotted out.

Mercifully, the role of the workhouse has disappeared. The buildings often became hospitals; many have now been given a new lease of life as smart flats, since time has lent glamour to buildings perceived a hundred years ago as little better than prisons.

In the 1940s, the UK government passed a series of Acts which established the welfare state: a guarantee of free basic care for everyone and a far cry from the dark days of the workhouse. Among the provisions made were free access to education for every child, a weekly allowance for children (now called 'child benefit'), a national insurance system, free health care and a system of benefits for people who were unemployed or in serious financial need.

One essential principle was the right to free care without the stigma of being on the receiving end of charity. As a result, we all know that if we fall ill or suffer a disastrous financial collapse, some kind of basic help will be available from the state and our families will not necessarily have to jump in to fill the breach.

In the rougher, tougher atmosphere of the 1980s and 1990s, many of these principles have seemed less secure than they once were. Benefits of all kinds have been given more grudgingly at the same time as state provision of hospitals and schools has been under serious threat of appearing second-rate by comparison with the services offered by private competitors. Even so, complete destitution is now unlikely and uncommon.

Another trend that is certain to affect your work includes the growing belief that institutional care robs people of dignity and that 'community care' is better. Many long-stay hospitals are being closed, and their clients moved to much smaller, more informal homes; there is a greater reluctance to admit elderly people to residential homes and a growing belief in the value of helping them live independently in their own homes for longer.

When you work as a professional carer it is easy to forget that, in spite of the increase in the need for paid care, the job you do is still the exception rather than the rule. Only three in every hundred elderly people live in residential care. In spite of the apparent 'selfishness' or inability to provide care of some families, up to 6 *million* people are caring unpaid for frail or handicapped relatives at home; the number of paid carers is at most only about one-twentieth of that. This considerable burden is carried by these 'informal carers' out of love and duty and by people often not fit, strong or well-off themselves. It is clearly a much more common response to the crisis of needing to provide care for another family member than handing them to the care of professionals.

Summary

This chapter has looked at why the need for professional carers has grown. Reasons explored include the fact that more people are living longer because of the dramatic rise in standards of living seen during the twentieth century as a result of increasing affluence, and improvements in food, contraception, medical care and public health. The growth of interest in preventive health care is also likely to increase longevity. At the same time as the number of older people has grown, the number of young people has fallen and family life itself is changing, with more frequent house moves, more divorce and more single-parent families. All these trends have tended to make it harder for families to care for their frailer members themselves, though many, of course, still do so.

2

Being a client

Why use the word 'client'?

If you are new to care support work, you might find it odd that the word 'client' is used to describe the people for whom you care, whether they are elderly people still living at home, people in day-care centres and sheltered housing, or younger people who are mentally and physically handicapped. At one training session for people new to the job, the tutor asked her group what words they normally used. Answers included 'inmate', 'patient', 'case', 'resident', 'guest' and 'my ladies and gentlemen'.

All these words have significantly different shades of meaning from 'client'. Ask yourself how you would feel about the use of these words in relation to yourself. 'Inmate' probably suggests that you are a prisoner, held in an institution against your will or as a punishment for some misdeed. 'Patient' suggest illness and also implies that you are expected to *be* patient and passive because a patient tends to be someone to whom things are done rather than someone who can actively take part in his or her own treatment. 'Case' suggests that you are a set of symptoms rather than an individual. Have you, for instance, ever been discussed in your presence by two doctors as if you were not there? Here is one client, now living in sheltered housing, but previously matron of a large urban hospital, recalling such an experience:

> I went to my doctor because I had a crusty discharge on both nipples. He trains other GPs so there was also a younger doctor there. I wasn't asked if I minded this though I probably would have been too intimidated to protest. They examined me then had a discussion while I lay there with no clothes on. 'Fascinating case,' said my GP, 'hope it isn't Paget's [disease]'.

'Yes', said the other one, 'that would be bad luck'. They ignored me completely. I suppose I was the one patient in a thousand who knew that 'Paget's' was a cancer, so I felt desperately worried and, later on, furious at their lack of sensitivity. Fortunately it wasn't cancer, but I changed to another GP in the same practice from that day on.

'Resident' is the most neutral of the words, but its disadvantage is that it can appear to define people completely by their roles as living in a particular place, something these clients object to strongly:

They speak of us as The Residents as if we were a football team. It implies that we're all the same. I don't like it – why label us at all?

I hate being call a 'resident'. It suggests I'll never leave, except feet first.

'Client' is now the word that most people in the caring professions prefer. The reason is that it is closely allied to the word 'customer'. As a customer in a shop you have the right to

- choose what to buy
- refuse to buy
- expect courteous, knowledgeable and prompt service
- complain
- go elsewhere if you are not satisfied

All this should be equally true of people who are receiving care – hence the word 'client', transferred from the vocabulary of other professional people who provide services, such as solicitors and accountants.

As recently as the 1960s, this philosophy would have seemed absurd to many carers. People who received care were, it was often implied, lucky to be getting it at all; it was hinted that they may even have been responsible for their own plight, so were expected to be grateful for what little they had. Here is one carer, now the proprietor of several highly successful and popular care homes, describing her first glimpse of the sort of place that was all too common even in the early 1960s:

I was doing a social work course and we were sent on visits

which we had to write up. One of mine was a geriatric hospital in London. One of the senior staff showed me round. I've never forgotten it. It was like a vision of hell: white walls, grey floors, two long rows of iron cots all with identical white bedspreads. The ward had about seventy such beds, each containing a very old, very frail person. You couldn't tell whether they were men or women as they all appeared to have wispy white hair and sunken yellow cheeks. They were just lying in bed dressed in grey shapeless garments, totally apathetic, waiting to die. I was only 21 at the time, but that's when I made up my mind that old age didn't have to be so dreadfully degrading and that I personally would go into this work to provide something better.

Fifteen years later I did! I have clients in my homes who are probably just as frail as the ones I saw so many years ago, but every one of them is treated as an individual. We guard their independence and mobility fiercely; hardly any of them is totally bedridden – we make sure of that!

Being dependent

Even though the word 'client' implies freedom to choose, in practice clients are people who depend on you for at least part of their care. How does this dependency affect their lives?

Restricted freedom to make decisions

Your clients will be individuals of widely different experience and personality. Probably the only thing that unites them is that they are all likely to have lost some of the freedoms to make decisions great and small that you take for granted. It is likely, for instance, that you can choose how you spend your leisure time. Most clients will have little choice on this point. For instance, even a client living in his or her own home may be restricted by disability to a narrow band of choices, as this severely disabled man describes:

> My life is all 'leisure', I suppose, because I can do so little for myself, but I can't drive, can't afford taxis, can't get to the library, can't shop, so how I spend my leisure comes down to reading the newspaper, listening to radio or watching TV. My home helps are great, but I'd love some other company

sometimes. I used to love going down the pub, but unless someone pushes me in my wheelchair, I'm stuck here.

This man's comments bring home that many clients have also lost the freedom to decide whom they live with and whom they see. They have restricted choices where friends are concerned. If they are living at home and have a telephone, they may be able to keep old friendships going, but if they have outlived all their old friends and family they will find it difficult to forge new friendships. A carer who visits you because she is paid to, can never provide the same kind of relationship as a friendship freely made between equals.

People who live in institutions have equally restricted freedoms as far as friendships are concerned. There may be visits to and from friends and family outside, but on admission to care, many clients are obliged to accept that their social circle from that point on is going to consist solely of other people in the home. These relationships can become intense – both rewarding and explosively antagonistic – a sign in both cases of the lack of freedom to walk away.

Equally, for many clients, there is no choice about where they live. If they are very frail, their families may have felt that they had to decide for them that such-and-such a home was best; some mentally handicapped clients may not be considered able enough to express a choice; sometimes there may simply not be a choice. Even when it comes to the actual rooms in which they live, clients may not have the freedom to make real decisions. Rooms may be decorated identically, bed covers may be the same colour, and only a few personal belongings may be allowed:

> We allow one chair and the equivalent of a suitcase of ornaments and so on. The rooms are very small. We just can't have too much clutter.

> What do patients have? Well . . . a locker, and by custom a chair in the day room which becomes 'theirs'.

Most of us like defining our personalities and interests not just by how we dress but also by how we decorate our homes. One person may like busy rooms, books, pictures and warm rusty colours, another may prefer clean white walls, bare of decorative detail. Some people like leaving a room cluttered, others are meticulously tidy. If you look after clients who live in their own homes, this freedom is one you can help them preserve. But clients in institutions, who may be allowed little more than a simple bedside locker, are often denied the basic human freedom to decorate and arrange their own personal space.

Many of the small daily freedoms that you take for granted will be denied your clients. You can decide what and when to eat, when to get up and when to go to bed, when to go to the lavatory, but can your clients do the same? However much choice is possible in theory, in practice do they have to wait for you to help them? One young woman client, who suffers from rheumatoid arthritis, describes her routine:

> I need my home help to get me out of bed and into bed. It takes about an hour by the time I've got washed, cleaned teeth, dressed, got to the loo and got out of bed because I'm so stiff and slow. I sometimes dream that the arthritis has gone and that I'm twelve again running upstairs screaming with laughter with my mum chasing me as a joke and getting under the bed to hide. Oh dear . . . it's many years since I could do that. I often think that being able to dress and undress at a time and pace I chose would be the best present of all.

This loss of health and mobility also takes away the freedom to make significant choices about the quality of life. A moving example was described by Elaine Heath, increasingly disabled by cerebral palsy. Paralysed and unable to speak, she can only communicate by operating an electric typewriter with her nose. She has three A levels, has taught herself Russian, has been married and divorced, and has been pregnant (and miscarried). In an interview in *The Independent* (3 October 1989) with Cherrill Hicks, she says her life has become not worth living since she became what she describes 'a social services project':

> In the mornings Elaine cannot get up before 9am – which is when her Care Assistant starts work. In the afternoons she must always be home at 4.30 – so that the Carer can take her to the lavatory before leaving for the day. (Even her bladder has to be regulated, she points out) . . . She can never go out and meet men; and after two close relationships, the prospect of staying single depresses her. 'I desperately want to love and be loved', she types with her nose. 'I'm terrified of growing old alone'.

Love and sex

Again, the freedom to choose to have a sex life may be more often denied than granted to your clients. Added to the overwhelming practical difficulties Elaine describes of actually getting out and meeting someone, is the unspoken assumption that somehow it is not seemly for elderly or physically dependent people to have the same sexual needs as the rest of us. A care officer with a voluntary organisation describes some of the difficulties this creates for her clients:

> We have a lot of young adult clients here. It's inevitable that romances and sexual relationships spring up, but a lot of the staff here seem to feel very uneasy about this. I remember one young couple, both in their early twenties, both severely physically disabled, who were determined that they were going to have a full sexual relationship. There was a tremendous fuss when the young man was discovered half-undressed in the young woman's room. Both sets of parents were brought in and everyone shook their heads and said the couple had to be responsible; they were told they shouldn't have intercourse because they couldn't manage contraception and if they had a baby, how on earth could they look after it? To their tremendous physical difficulties of actually *managing* any kind of sexual act was added the awful indignity of other people pompously telling them they didn't have a right to even think of it. Actually, what they needed was someone to help them both get undressed and get into bed then to leave them to it!

This kind of control, often justified by managers as being 'cruel to be kind' robs clients of the right to take decisions and to take risks on exactly the same basis as everyone else. Being old, being disabled, being ill, does not mean that you stop thinking about sex or being capable of a full sexual relationship. Indeed, recent research shows that interest in sex and normal sexual activity can and do continue into very old age.

Lack of privacy

Privacy for intimate tasks, privacy to do what you like, privacy to be alone in a space that cannot be entered without permission . . . these are all important and basic human needs. Some of your clients may find their lack of privacy the most painful of all the psychological adjustments that need to be made when on the receiving end of care. Intimate tasks like wiping their bottom may have to be surrendered to other people; perhaps some of them can no longer do simple tasks such as cutting their toenails, and even this is potentially humiliating, described here with furious resentment by one client:

> I've always had a 'thing' about my feet, I've got corns, bunions and horrible horny misshapen nails on most of my toes, but until now they've been my personal problem. I still feel a wave of real shame when my home carer cuts my nails for me, but I know I can't do them myself, so I've just got to put up with it. It's as much as I can do to stay polite – I feel like snapping and snarling I hate it so much. I don't *want* someone else cutting my nails.

These necessary physical tasks can be as difficult for the carer as the cared-for, but carers can often forget that a client's privacy can be invaded in other, more subtle ways. Here is a middle-aged son describing the problems his father had in coming to terms with the need for help in his home:

> It was obvious he couldn't struggle on totally alone, and it was keeping the house clean that really bothered him. I suggested getting a friendly neighbour in who'd offered to help, paid, with housework, but he said no, she'd tell everyone his business, for instance, how many cups and saucers he had and how many were cracked! So I said, well what about a home help? and he said oh no, that would be even worse because she'd be going into other people's houses too, telling them *his* business. Ridiculously illogical though it seems, he was actually prepared to contemplate going into a residential home rather than have an unwelcome visitor in his own home . . .!

The same feeling is described by a meals-on-wheels worker:

> One client insists that I stay on his front door step. I've never yet been inside his home, after seven years! Once or twice, he's been ill, but even then it's been the same routine. He makes it very clear that it's his home and his privacy; I have to respect that – I think I might feel the same in his circumstances.

At least these clients were still in their own homes, so they could still guard their privacy to a great extent. Although many homes are now sensitive to the need to provide somewhere totally private for residents, you may still find establishments where, for instance, staff do not knock before entering a client's room. This behaviour can only be seen as an intrusion, but it is based on the idea that the room belongs to the proprietor or local authority rather than to the client.

Loss of dignity

Being dependent on other people's care can very easily rob you of dignity. It is potentially humiliating to have to ask to be taken to the lavatory, to need to be fed with a spoon, to be unable to speak even when your brain is still functioning perfectly normally, to be talked about in your presence without your opinion being asked . . . all these things take away dignity. This is a problem which crops up more in long-term residential care than it does for patients in hospitals or for frail people still living in their own homes. The key difference seems to be that in hospitals patients are assumed to be on their way home. It is acknowledged that they have a life outside the hospital to which they will return, and this gives them power. People who live permanently in institutions have no home other than the institution. It is widely assumed that only the absolutely desperate would opt for residential care; therefore they become objects of pity, and to be pitied is to suffer loss of dignity, a feeling vividly described here by an elderly client living in a nursing home:

> I feel people are thinking, well *she* must have been a right old cow, otherwise why isn't she living with her daughter? You only feel half a person once you end up here. You've been abandoned . . . and everybody knows it.

Which comes first – losing your dignity or being patronized? It's difficult to say, but the two are certainly closely linked.

Lack of money

Most of your clients are likely not to be well off. Being disabled, being old, being mentally ill affects their standard of living. Their disability, frailty or illness makes it difficult to earn a living. And they will incur additional costs as a result of their condition. Elizabeth, a woman with severe arthritis, considers herself lucky, because she's still able to work, but it is clear that her standard of living has been considerably reduced by her disability:

> The only kind of work I can do is the sort where travelling is minimal, and even so, I have to have a car to get to work as I just can't manage public transport. My car has to be an automatic with power steering – my wrists and ankles are too feeble to cope with a 'normal' car, and that costs a lot more. I've had to pay privately for two joint replacement operations, because I was by then so lame that I'd have lost my job if I'd waited the three years I was quoted for an NHS one, so I borrowed the money from the bank. I can't wear shop-bought clothes because I have such swollen limbs, so I have to have everything made for me; needless to say, this is much more expensive than buying things at Marks & Spencer. I've got to have help at home because there's no way I can do housework that involves lifting and bending. I'm lucky really that my paid work doesn't depend on physical strength, otherwise I'd have been unemployed and living in dire poverty for years. As it is, I've just about kept going. I'm really lucky that I have an Orange Badge for my car, but unfortunately I don't qualify for any extra financial help.

Many frail and dependent people cannot work, and their benefits do not cover the considerable extra costs incurred by their condition. One home care assistant describes here how this affects one of her clients:

> Peter is severely handicapped and is cared for by his sister. He is doubly incontinent, partially paralysed and cannot speak or feed himself. He dribbles constantly. The laundry bill for their house is enormous; they get through washing machines and sheets and duvets at a phenomenal rate. He needs incontinence pads, of course, and his clothing has to be replaced far more often than is the case for 'normal' people. He cannot read but loves television, so his sister keeps him well supplied with videos, even though they can't really afford it. They get allowances, of course, but this can't come anywhere near meeting the real costs.

Lack of money also cuts down the range of other choices open to clients. Those who are very poor are likely to have to depend on 'free' services rather than paying for and choosing their own carer. This in itself, makes it more difficult for them to complain about the quality of the service they receive. Although some kinds of leisure activities do not cost money, many do; holidays, day trips, visits to restaurants, sport and hobbies could all be beyond the means of those whose only source of income is state benefits.

Several surveys have shown how far behind most disabled people lag financially. One such survey suggested that the typical income of a disabled person was only about one-third of the national average. So again, lack of money is likely to mean lack of choice, often with little prospect of an improvement in financial circumstances. This woman, now in her late sixties and living independently, finds it difficult to adjust to the idea of permanent poverty:

> My heart condition means that I now get puffed and tired very easily. Previously, I used to do some sewing here – I dressed dolls for a local wholesaler. It was badly paid, but at least it gave me a bit of extra cash and I used to meet a few people when they delivered and collected the dolls and fabric and so on.
>
> I'm completely dependent now on my pension. If I didn't see my home help I'd hardly see anyone because I can't get out. I can't afford taxis and can't manage buses. The walk from the bus stop is uphill on the way back and it's too much. I find it difficult to accept that there's nothing I can do to improve my financial situation because I'm just not well enough to work, but nor am I ill enough to qualify for any other benefits.

Institutions and their effects on clients

So the word 'client' is not just a fashionable label. Its use sums up a whole philosophy of care. But although this may be the ideal, in practice many of the people who receive care are not treated as clients but as 'patients' or 'inmates'. The result is that they can very quickly lose their ability to act independently. You may perhaps have had some personal experience of this if you or people close to you have had a spell in hospital, as happened to this care assistant and her husband:

My husband went into hospital two years ago to have a medical problem properly investigated. As soon as he arrived he was asked to undress and get into bed; I never knew why – he wasn't actually ill. From that moment on, a thirty-two-year-old professional man used to making decisions and managing other people became like a little lost boy. They gave him a new drug that made him nauseous, but he wouldn't complain – I had to do it for him. Within a few days it was no use my bringing him office gossip – he just wasn't interested. What happened on the ward, what the other patients said and did was much more important. I suggested one evening that he got dressed and came down to the pub around the corner with me. He looked quite shocked and said he'd have to ask Sister first. I pointed out that he was perfectly free to leave the ward and could tell the staff where he was going without asking permission, and he looked quite surprised! I was appalled that he seemed to shed his individuality and confidence so quickly. This incident gave me real insight into the behaviour of the people I care for in my job.

At its most extreme, when people have lived in institutions for many years, whether children's homes, hospitals or care homes, they can very quickly fall into institutionalised behaviour. Severely institutionalized people have lost all their self-esteem and so cannot make even the simplest choices. They lose the ability to have conversations or to form friendships. They certainly don't have the self-confidence to question the quality of their care. Here is one care worker, working in a long-stay hospital for the mentally ill, talking about Pearl, a woman in her sixties who has been in hospital for forty years. Her original hospital records have been lost, but Pearl thinks that the reason she was admitted was that she was suffering from acute depression:

Pearl is very frightened by having to make decisions, so we are helping her to learn how to do this in a series of small ways. Does she prefer to wear her red dress or her blue one? Would she like to sit next to Mary at lunchtime or next to Pat? She thinks so little of herself that she can't *start* a conversation with anyone and if you speak to her, she doesn't look at you, she looks past you or at the floor. The little money she has has been handled for her for so many years that she's terrified of shops, so we go out on trips to buy small things. Now she's able to hand over the money on her own, but this is a new achievement – previously she expected me to do it for her. She still can't actually speak to a shop assistant.

If you work with elderly clients in a residential home, you may have seen similar behaviour, even if it is not quite so extreme as in this case:

All our old people sit around in their chairs in the lounge all day long. A lot of them are quite able-bodied so they could go out into the town, but they don't seem to want to. Some of them just spend hours staring into space or sleeping. All they want to know is how long it is till lunch or supper – some of them can't even be bothered to look at their own watches.

It is important to point out that staff can become institutionalized, too, although in a slightly different way; only able to operate through rules and regulations, and also finding it difficult to make decisions for themselves. One auxiliary describes the effect on him of working in such an environment:

I worked in a long-stay mental hospital. It was run on very old-fashioned lines with patients heavily drugged to keep them quiet and a rigid system of reward and punishments (a *lot* of punishments). I had absolutely no discretion to treat patients as I thought fit; it was care by numbers. There were times of the day and week for everything and woe betide you if you departed from it. In the end I became like a robot, I lost faith in my ability to decide anything on my own. I realized I had to get out because it was affecting my personal life, too.

Why do people become dependent?

Clients and staff who become institutionalized and dependent have learnt to behave in this way. It happens because the institution is run for the benefit of the system, not of the clients. You can still, for instance, find some hospitals which have lights out at 9.30 p.m. and wake patients as early as 5.00 a.m., far earlier than most people either go to sleep or wake naturally. The reason is that it suits the shift pattern of the staff, not that it suits the needs of the patients. Realizing this, many hospitals now leave patients to sleep and wake in their own time, without any collapse of hospital routines.

This is just one small example of how systems can develop which suit the institution but which destroy the individuality of the client as well as the ability of staff to make decisions relating to their care. Here are some others, along with the arguments often used to justify such actions:

Clients' clothes are chosen by staff	'It's quicker, and they don't mind'
Clients are discouraged from doing anything risky	'We have to make sure they're safe – we're the ones who get the blame if anything goes wrong'
Staff don't knock before entering clients' rooms Everyone eats the same food at the same time	'This is the only way we can cope; it isn't a hotel, you know'
Clients and their relatives are not involved in discussions and decisions about their care and are not encouraged to question its quality	'They wouldn't understand'
Clients' money is kept for them; they have to ask if they want it	'It might get stolen'
Clients are discouraged from having their own furniture and other possessions	'Other people might get jealous – we like everyone to be the same' 'It's easier to keep the room clean'
Entertainment and leisure activities are compulsory – clients can't opt out unless actually ill	'It's only fair to the people putting on the event'
It is assumed that clients do not have sexual needs	'It would upset everyone if people had love affairs'

Underlying all the justifications offered for these actions are two assumptions. One is that everyone is the same, so it is all right to treat them in the same way – for instance, by making them all go to bed or wake up at the same time. Clearly we are not all the same. You are bound to know people who are happily pottering about at 1 o'clock in the morning and others who are always up at dawn; some who like ten hours' sleep and others who rarely have more than five. We do not suddenly become uniform in our preferences just because we live in an institution. So the assumption that everyone can be treated in the same way is false.

The other assumption is that people in institutions are less grown-up than the rest of us. It is all right for us to choose to wear an outfit others think peculiar, to embark on a friendship that others think risky, or to leave a purse on top of a shopping bag where it might get stolen, but it is not all right for clients. The problem with this argument is that, unfortunately, if you treat people as if they are child-like for long enough, that is indeed how they become. The key point about adult, responsible behaviour is having power and control over your life. When that is taken away it robs people of their confidence and self-esteem. This client spent three weeks in respite care in a residential home while the son who normally cares for her went on holiday. She still thinks of it with horror:

> I have multiple sclerosis so I'm in a wheelchair, but that doesn't mean I'm a dummy. I was treated as if I wasn't there a lot of the time and talked about as 'we'. How are *we* today? Are *we* ready for a little drink? At first I fought against it and gave sarcastic replies, but they just looked hurt and I heard one say to another: 'Goodness, we *are* a difficult lady, aren't we?' In the end I knuckled under and behaved like the passive doll they wanted. I *despised* myself for doing it and it took me a long time to get my confidence back. I even found it difficult to make phone calls once I was back at home because I hadn't been able to use the phone when I was away, except with huge difficulty, and I caught myself thinking, who would want to talk to a nobody like me?

It would be quite wrong to suggest that care support workers encourage dependency for sinister reasons. Most often it is done for the very best and kindest of motives, but it needs to be challenged. Not only does it take away the basic right to independence which we all have, it also potentially takes away a lot of the satisfaction which the work provides. After all, the 'passive doll' quoted in the story above would be a lot less rewarding to look after than the sprightly, interesting woman she normally was.

What do clients need?

In many ways the question 'what do clients need?' is a bogus one. The reason is that what you need and what your clients need is fundamentally the same. The great psychologist, Abraham Maslow, produced a famous analysis of 'human need', which is normally drawn as a pyramid. At its base are the fundamental needs just to survive. When these are met, the next most fundamental need is to be secure – to know, for instance, that you have enough money to meet your bills and feed yourself. Next is the need to love and be loved and admired. Nearly at the top of the pyramid is the need to achieve – to feel proud of what you do. Finally, at the very top, is the need to serve other people, to feel useful.

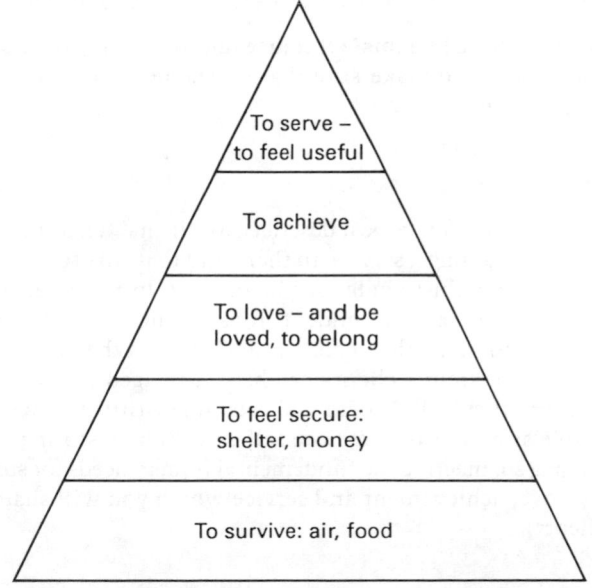

Figure 1 Maslow's pyramid: the hierarchy of human needs

You may feel that you cannot even tick off all the items on this list of 'needs' for yourself. If, for instance, you are in the middle of a divorce, you may feel that your need to love and be loved is not being met. Maybe you are also hard up and are worried about whether your salary can keep pace with inflation. However, the chances are that as a carer you are more likely to be in a position to have all your needs met than are your clients. For instance, you know that in your own job you are supplying an essential service. Because of their dependency, many of your clients would only be able to say that their need to survive was being met; they may not even feel secure because of their financial worries. Where the need for affection is concerned, many of your clients may have no one to give them affection or admiration. Fewer still will be able to feel that there is anything they can achieve, and hardly any would be able to say that they are 'useful':

> Our clients in this home lead really pathetic lives. What's for dinner is their only interest. There are very few who are actually confused or very frail, but they have no real friends, their families only visit rarely. The boredom and sameness of their day really just emphasizes that they are waiting to die.

Does it have to be like this? Of course not. As a carer, an important part of your job is to make sure that *all* the needs in the pyramid can be met, however simply.

Summary

The people you care for are best described as 'clients'. This emphasizes that you are providing a service to them and that this service is one they have every right to judge for its quality. In practice, the fact that your clients are dependent robs them of many of the opportunities to make the decisions and choices that you take for granted. At its extreme, clients can be so damaged by this process that they lose their self-esteem and become institutionalized. Part of your role as a carer is to restore self-esteem by restoring choice, and, in doing so, meeting the fundamental human needs for survival, security, love, achievement and service which you will share with your clients.

3

The fundamentals of caring

Being a client is not a comfortable or enviable position. To help clients, there are certain basic principles of caring which should filter into every aspect of your work with them. This chapter explores these principles and looks at some of the ways you could consider using them in all your dealings with clients.

Encouraging independence

Clients are people who have been making decisions for themselves all their lives. If they have not been doing so – for example, severely institutionalized clients who have been living in long-stay hospitals – then part of your work will be to help them relearn independence. The decisions clients make may not be the ones you would make. For instance, you may think their choice of clothing in poor taste: you would not choose such a dress or jacket yourself. But if that is the client's choice, then that is the one you must go along with.

In the long run, it will be a help to you if you encourage independence in clients. You will feel less burdened by responsibility for them in areas where in fact it is neither your right nor your duty to feel responsible; clients will retain the ability to do things for themselves, thus freeing you to give your time to people whose physical or mental frailty does mean that you have to perform many tasks for them.

As far as possible, clients should go on living the same kind of lives that they have enjoyed previously. Old age, residential living or dependence on social services help should not in themselves mean that people lose their right to choice. In practice, this can be difficult to achieve:

Mr Stevens is eighty-three and has just moved into our care home because his health has deteriorated to the point where he cannot look after himself alone. His daughter, who did look after him, has had to move away. He worked in agriculture as a salesman and all his life has got up at 5.30 a.m. 'because farm life starts early'. He needs help in getting out of bed and getting dressed. Our shift system means that it's really inconvenient to find someone to help him so early. It suits us much better to get everyone up at around 7.30 to 8.00. But Mr Stevens is fretting and upset. He says he lies awake and gets depressed because he can't get up.

What is to be done about the plight of Mr Stevens? He has had a lifetime of getting up early and wishes to continue to do so. It is inconvenient for the staff who are busy with a shift-change and prefer their existing pattern where the day staff get clients up and breakfast is served at 8.30 a.m. Here there is a straight clash between the clearly stated needs of the client and the needs of the institution. Mr Stevens is lucky; he is living in a home where the clients' needs are taken seriously. The solution to his dilemma has been to negotiate a compromise. A care assistant comes in at 6.00 a.m., helps him get up and makes him a cup of tea. He postpones shaving and dressing until later, when one of the day staff helps him. Both he and his carers are happy with this solution.

Encouraging acceptable risks

One of the reasons why you may find yourself resisting the idea of encouraging independence in clients is that risk-taking and independence go hand in hand, and risk-taking can pose some uncomfortable dilemmas for carers. Here are some examples:

Ellie is a wheelchair-bound twenty-seven-year-old living in a specially adapted one-storey extension to her parents' house. She has not come to terms with the partial paralysis resulting from a road accident a year ago. Daily visits from a home care assistant give her parents valuable respite from caring for her round the clock. Until now, Ellie has been content to have meals, tea and coffee prepared for her. Now she is beginning to feel less depressed and is keen to start cooking for herself.

Her parents say her hands are far too weak to hold cooking pots and that even tea-making is out of the question because of the risk of scalding herself. Her care assistant thinks that Ellie should be allowed to start simple cooking, as greater independence is the key to her recovery.

Leonard has always been a keen gardener: it is his main hobby and he has a large, well-cultivated garden. Now he is in his late seventies and has experienced several falls and two blackouts, all of which happened while gardening. His home help is concerned: she feels that he ought to give up his garden.

Mrs Barrett has brittle bones and has had several falls. Two of them involved fractures and resulted in long stays in hospital. Now she is so nervous of walking that she is spending long hours sitting in a chair and when she does walk, will only shuffle along slowly, using a frame. Her doctor's opinion is that immobility poses greater medical risks than walking. Her home care assistant is meeting serious resistance to this idea from Mrs Barrett.

John and Sarah are both mentally handicapped young adults. Sarah's handicap is more profound than John's. They now live in a hostel with a small group of similar clients. An emotional relationship is developing between them. Staff worry that it may become a full sexual relationship. They do not feel that Sarah can understand the implications of this and say that a pregnancy would have a destructive effect on her already fragile stability.

In these examples we can see some of the complexity of encouraging or discouraging risk-taking in clients. There may be pressure from the client to take the risk – for instance, to go on gardening, or to have a relationship – which you may feel is unwise and risks compromising the client's health, safety or emotional well-being. There may be pressure from the client to be independent – for instance, to make her own tea – which is opposed by the clients' family, but encouraged by the carer. Then there is the case where the client is content to allow her independence to slip away because she is frightened of taking risks. Mrs Barrett's carers feel that she should be encouraged to take *more* risks in the interests both of her long-term health and of discouraging her dependence on care from others. In some cases, the carers will try to limit risky behaviour because they fear prosecution or reproaches from the client's family if something goes wrong.

No such case is ever simple but some rough rules of thumb can help. First, you need the hard, impartial information that will help you to assess the risk coolly. How strong are Ellie's arms and hands? Are they likely to become stronger if she had physiotherapy and exercised them regularly? What can she grip firmly? Has anyone watched her, ready to help and supervise if necessary, while she fills a kettle, boils it and makes tea? If so, how well did she manage? Going through a calm and orderly assessment of the problem from this point of view will have many benefits. It will give everyone involved a better base from which to make the decision. If Ellie really can manage the tea-making on her own then proving it will help convince you and her parents that she should be allowed to carry on. If there are difficulties, then these may be sufficient to show Ellie herself that she ought to continue to receive help – maybe just with some aspects of the tasks or until she recovers more strength in her hands.

The next step is to look at how colleagues and clients have handled similar problems in the past. You may perhaps have staff meetings where this kind of issue can be discussed; your employer may have a policy on such matters which will help. Your immediate boss is certain to know of other cases where decisions were reached which could help you and your client in various ways. These discussions will give you guidance on how other people found solutions to similar problems. Consulting colleagues and the clients' family will also help you come to a better decision with the client because everyone will have discussed the problem and agreed a solution. This is always better than one person making a decision alone, especially where it involves the welfare of others.

Finally, and most importantly, you can look for ways to negotiate so that you still allow the client the chance to be independent, but you reduce the most worrying risks. For instance, Mrs Barrett's carers could agree with her that she increases the total amount of walking that she does, that she uses a stick and not a frame, but that she will do this at first with a care assistant constantly at her side. Leonard might be persuaded to confine most of his gardening to the hours when his home help is in his house so that prompt assistance is always nearby. John and Sarah could be given intensive help; the assessment in John's case might conclude that he was capable of understanding and using contraception. If not, then some suitable contraceptive method might be devised for Sarah.

Sometimes, of course, the risks to the client's health outweigh the gains of independence. Here is a case in point:

> Mr and Mrs Laxton live in a pleasant suburban area. Mrs Laxton has developed Alzheimer's disease and is becoming increasingly confused. Mr Laxton has diabetes which has affected his sight and his kidneys. None the less, he has devotedly looked after his wife with the help of neighbours and a home care assistant who calls four times a week. Now that Mr Laxton is having to make more frequent visits to hospital as a day patient, it is proving impossible to cover all his absences. His wife has several times been brought home by neighbours or the police because she has been found wandering in the streets wearing a nightdress. She often cannot remember her name or where she lives. On her own in the house she has twice left on an unlit gas tap. Mr Laxton believes he can carry on looking after his wife, but it is clear that the stress of her situation is also affecting his own frail health.

In this situation, the assessment by the GP and social services in consultation with her carer all pointed to the need for institutional care for his wife. The deterioration in her condition was so rapid that she was becoming a danger to herself and to others. She was admitted to the geriatric unit of a local hospital.

However, we should be wary of thinking that 'solving' a problem through admission to care is always 'right'. In Mrs Laxton's case no doubt it was. But in many cases this produces misery for the client. Research quoted by Alison Norman in her excellent book, *Rights and Risk*, points to evidence suggesting that a quarter of the confused patients admitted to one psychiatric hospital had died within three weeks of admission. She also quotes a study showing that in many cases old people are less safe in care than outside it, with a very high percentage of total falls occurring in institutional homes. She comments:

> If avoidance of risk is indeed a prime objective, moving people out of their homes may not be the best way of achieving it,

and that the more they appear to be at risk where they are, the worse will be that prognosis if they are moved.

Encouraging self-esteem

We have already seen in Chapter 2 that being dependent on others for care can rob people of self-esteem. Some clients may never have had self-esteem:

> Patrick was damaged by the drug thalidomide which his mother took during pregnancy. He was born without arms or legs. His parents felt ashamed of his disability which they constantly referred to as 'gross deformity'. They encouraged him to hide from social contact and he did badly at school, in spite of his above-average intelligence. He now lives in a hostel but is unpopular with other clients because of his destructive behaviour and sarcastic tongue.

> Tracy was sexually abused by both her parents. She ran away from home at age twelve, and had a baby at thirteen. The baby was adopted and Tracy was taken into care. Tracy's parents were eventually prosecuted and imprisoned – something for which Tracy quite wrongly blames herself. By eighteen she had had two long spells as a voluntary patient in a psychiatric hospital and is now living in a half-way house. She refers to herself as 'a little slag, a little no-good'.

If you are working as a carer with clients like Patrick and Tracy, part of your job will be to help them learn the self-esteem that the neglect and abuse of their parents has denied them. For others, it is not so much a lifetime of deprivation as their recent experience which has been hurtful. Illness, bereavement, divorce or sudden poverty may all have produced the sorts of dramatic changes in clients' lives which make them feel lesser people than they once were. Here is how two such clients describe their own reactions to events of this sort:

> I didn't marry till I was in my late thirties and I absolutely idolized my husband. He was everything to me. When we were in our sixties he shattered me by announcing that he was leaving me for someone he'd met at our local pub. I couldn't believe it; I'd always thought we were happy. The effect on

> me has been terrible. The humiliation of everyone knowing was awful for a start, then I suddenly had a lot less money, so I couldn't buy nice clothes any more. Now I've had a stroke and my face looks funny all down one side. I feel like a non-person.
>
> I always said I'd kill myself before allowing myself to move into an old people's home. Well, perhaps I will. Only people who've lost hope come here, don't they? People that everyone has agreed are surplus to requirements . . . people waiting to die.

For most of us, our self-esteem is closely linked to the image we like to present to the world. This may be connected to external things like clothes or other possessions, to how we wear our hair, to the income we have or to the relationships we are proud to claim. Having a job may be especially important because it is proof that someone thinks highly enough of you to put a price on your abilities. In a competitive and materialistic society like ours, not to have a job (whether because of your age, your health, or some other reason) often makes people feel that they must therefore not have a worth.

Enhancing clients' self-esteem can affect all your dealings with them. For instance, show them that you value their opinions and feelings. Ask how they like to be addressed, whether by first name or by title, and stick to their preference. Ask what they think of the day's local, national and international news, ask them what they think of whatever is going on in their street or the home. Show by your replies that you know they are equals. Ask how they prefer to be shaved, fed or dressed; ask what clothes they would like to wear and stick to their preferences; do not impose your own.

Another useful way of building self-esteem is to notice and praise every achievement, however small. Here is a physiotherapist specializing in work with older people, talking about how and why she does this:

> In my work, many of my clients can often only make tiny improvements, if any. Even so, a lot of my energy goes into remembering what they could do in the previous session and praising even the most minute change. It's so important, I feel it's the only way people are going to get movement back into damaged tissue because they feel 'I really achieved something there – good on me!'.

Finally, it is important to give clients the chance to talk about their previous achievements. In this way they can recapture some of the pride they felt in the past, as well as knowing that recounting such events still has the power to impress others. All good care assistants will find dozens of ways to do this. Here are some of them:

> We published a little booklet of wartime reminiscences. Great fun! Several people were interviewed for the local radio and newspaper – did their confidence a world of good to be taken so seriously.

> When people have had the chance to read the newspapers I deliberately look for ways to ask people about things that were different when they were young so that they can have a little boast if they want to.

> Looking back on family life is always a good way of reminiscing in a positive way. I tell clients about some of my current family problems, and ask their advice. It's surprising what they come up with – some of them have some pretty racy stories to tell and a lot of them are very wise – they've really helped me.

Protecting privacy

Everyone has the right to some space and time which is completely private. Needing care puts your clients' right to privacy in jeopardy. For instance, in some residential homes people may have single rooms, but staff may walk in without knocking. Yet in such homes there is often a staff area which is labelled 'private' and clients are not allowed to enter without permission. Clients' bathrooms and lavatories may not have locks, while staff lavatories do. For home care assistants the danger is more subtle. You know you are in someone else's home, so your behaviour is probably more delicate – for instance, you probably always knock on the front door, even if you have a key, but does that give you permission to go anywhere in the client's house? Does it mean you clean the house in the same way that you would clean your own?

> I never, ever, assume that it's OK to go into a bedroom without asking. Even where I've worked with a client for years, I always say: 'OK to do the bedroom now?' In the same way, if I need to use the loo myself, I always say where I'm going – I don't assume.

When I visit a client for the first time I always discuss what rules they feel happy with. For instance, do they want me to ask every time I use the kitchen to make tea? Are they happy for me to go anywhere in the house, or are there some parts that are out of bounds? Can I open chests of drawers or not? When I've been a few times, I make sure we have the discussion again. It's very easy to cause offence without meaning to.

The risk in care work is that efficiency and the urge to save time can get in the way of the client's need for privacy. It may be quicker to vacuum clean several rooms at once from one long lead, leaving all the doors open, but doing so exposes clients to the feeling that their privacy has been lost, because any passer-by can see in. It is easy to assume that your own way of cleaning a house, perhaps starting from the top and working down, is the way a client would also like it done, but how do you know, unless you ask? It is easy to assume that a client whose home is dirty and smelly will be grateful for your disinfectant and broom, but if getting it clean involves disturbing her treasured collection of old clothes, can you be certain that it is better to be clean than to have left her clothes undisturbed and her privacy untouched?

Certain sensible rules apply to all your dealings with clients because preserving their privacy is always likely to be an issue, given the nature of your work:

- Knock before going into a client's room.
- Ask permission before you disturb a client's possessions in any way.
- Ask how clients would like their rooms cleaned and tidied.
- Shut doors and draw curtains before washing and toileting clients.
- Keep clients covered by using sheets wherever possible to preserve dignity during washing and toileting.
- Medical treatment should be possible without always having a carer present.
- It should always be possible for telephone calls to be made in private without the risk of being overheard.
- Letters and personal documents should be considered sacrosanct. You should not read them unless invited to and in such cases you should not divulge their contents to others.

Preserving confidentiality

Your work as a carer will often mean that you know a lot about clients'
private lives. They or their families may share confidential information with you, or you may need to know confidential details about
your clients in order to be fully involved in their care. Such information can be dynamite and sharing it inappropriately can cause tremendous damage because it leads to rumours and gossip which may
permanently affect clients' lives:

> We admitted an elderly single man who had been very ill, but
> was making a reasonable recovery. He took a long time to settle
> in and one of the other residents asked me what was wrong
> with him. To my eternal shame, I told her that he'd had an
> unusual kind of pneumonia and had lost a lot of weight.
>
> Within a day, I really mean a day, it was right round the home
> that he had AIDS and all the other residents were boycotting
> him. Two of the staff threatened to resign because they didn't
> want to deal with him. It wasn't true at all that he had AIDS
> but someone had put two and two together and made five
> because of the symptoms I'd described. The rumour was traced
> back to me and I was disciplined. The client was very, very
> unhappy and upset. I had made a situation that was already
> difficult for him far worse. It all died down eventually, but it
> took several months. It still makes me prickle all over to think
> of it.

Although, as this description shows, the need for confidentiality
is crucial, the trend in care work is towards people working as a team.
This means that several people may now need to have information
that was previously possessed by only one or two.

It is difficult to set down strict rules about confidentiality, but some
basic principles are:

- Find out what the practice of your own employers is and whether
  they have a policy on confidentiality.
- Never tell people outside work or other clients any details of a
  client's life and circumstances, whatever the temptation; most
  people find it hard not to pass on interesting gossip but if the gossip
  circulates it could damage both your client and you.
- Always ask yourself whether a colleague or member of another
  team really needs to share the information to help the client.

- Ask yourself whether you really need to know confidential details of a client's life or whether you are just curious.
- If you don't have the client's permission to share the information, think carefully before you pass it on, even to a colleague.
- Make sure that clients know the outcome of confidential discussions that the care team have about them.
- Let clients see their own records wherever possible; this discourages everyone on the care staff from writing patronizing and inaccurate comments.
- Establish the legal position – for instance, if a client tells you that another carer is sexually abusing her, what is the law on this point and what is your responsibility?
- Do not be afraid to consult your manager, telling your client that you are doing so, when it is clear that you cannot solve a problem of confidentiality on your own.

Respecting individuality

If you have only ever lived in one community and led one kind of life, mixing with one kind of person, it can come as a shock to find yourself confronted as a carer with all the rich variety of human society that care work can involve. This carer speaks for many when she describes the shock and challenge this meant for her:

> I was brought up in a nice, neat Nottingham suburb on an estate where everyone lived in the same kind of house, had the same kind of job with the same kind of income, and had the same kinds of opinion. When I married I moved to London and when my children were at school, I started working as a home carer. I was immediately mixing with people from all races, cultures and religions, people with very different beliefs and values from my own; people who sometimes thought that English society represented total immorality and hated having to receive 'charity' from it. For example, I worked with people from India who had quite different standards of hygiene – who thought, for instance, that having a bath was a truly disgusting process because it involved wallowing in dirty water and only a shower got you really clean. Some of my clients were Muslim women and I found it fairly hard to accept the restricted role

that their religion and culture appears to box them into. At first, my thought was 'Why aren't they like me?' meaning 'They *should be* like me'. But I gradually came to realize that people's language, religion, dress and everything else is part of what makes them individuals, and that it's not my business as a carer to challenge any of that. It's been difficult, though, shedding those suburban prejudices!

As this carer has discovered, it has to be part of your professional mental equipment that you can accept every client as an individual, whose race, culture and language may be different from your own. In practice this means understanding that clients may lead lives and have preferences which are quite unlike your own, and that is their right.

For instance, they may have a different religion whose observance makes significant differences to their daily lives. Foods that you enjoy may be forbidden to them. Muslims do not eat pork, nor do Jews. Jews may 'keep kosher', that is they observe certain strict rules of food hygiene. Hindus do not eat beef. Fasting, linked to religious festivals, is an important feature of many religions. Especially for the older generations in ethnic minority communities, social customs may be very different from your own. For instance, it is considered immodest for a Muslim woman to look directly at a man she does not know; there may be traditional ways in which it is acceptable to dress and which, if breached, will cause great distress.

When a substantial new wave of people from other countries first came to Britain after 1945, it was often assumed that such people 'must' learn English if it was not their first language. Of course, many did; their children are often bilingual, and their grandchildren may not speak or understand their grandparents' mother tongue at all, they may only speak English. But many of the older generation, particularly the women, remained isolated from English neighbours, with few chances to learn the language. Now that they are old and many of them are in need of care, they can be at enormous psychological disadvantage if they are also perceived as somehow 'handicapped' and lesser people because they are speaking another language. A client's own language is a basic right and an important part of their culture.

So, too, is sexuality. As long as its expression does not break the law, it is not appropriate for carers to do any more than to accept the client's choice. Here another carer describes a challenge to her previously set ideas:

> Of course I knew about homosexuality, but I'd always thought that gay people were limp-wristed joke figures. I was really surprised when one of my cases, Walter, turned out to be one partner in a gay relationship. He'd got Parkinson's disease and his partner, Sydney, couldn't really go on coping with him alone. I was amazed to discover that they'd lived quietly together for about 40 years and were so *ordinary*. Even so, at first I found the double bed slightly worrying but it was funny how quickly I came to terms with it. In the end I came to admire the quality and depth of their loyalty to each other which would have put many 'normal' couples to shame.

One good reason for accepting a client's individuality is that you cannot change it anyway. You are not living their lives for them and you can waste a lot of time and energy trying to get them to conform to your rules. Your client likes cats, owns two, and her flat is cluttered with empty cat-food tins and full cat-litter trays; the place definitely smells a little unpleasant. You may be able to clean the litter trays, wash the floor and throw away the tins, but are you really likely to be able to change your client's mind about liking cats? Of course not. Equally importantly, her feelings about cats are her business, not yours. If she doesn't notice the smell, perhaps it shouldn't worry you too much, as long as you feel you can keep the worst of the health risks at bay. Would it have been appropriate for the home carer just quoted to give Walter and his partner a moral lecture? Of course not. Not only would it have been a total waste of time, it would also have been offensive.

Sometimes you may be faced with the reverse problem; you may be rejected or attacked by the client on the grounds that you are the 'wrong' race, religion or sex. Behaving assertively (see page 149) is the only way to deal with these unpleasant situations. Putting up with racist comments (a passive response) or exchanging insults (an aggressive response) are not suitable tactics. Remaining calm, courteous and stating the sort of behaviour you expect from the client is the only possible way to deal with the situation:

> I was assigned a very difficult elderly white couple, both in very poor health. The moment the door was opened I knew

there would be problems. The man immediately said: 'We don't want no darkie helping us – you can tell the social [services] that we want an English person'. I held my ground and stayed very polite, though I was boiling inside, and explained that my role was to help them and why didn't we go inside to discuss it. Very reluctantly they did let me in. I said I was an English person, born and bred on Merseyside and described what I could do for them. They calmed down when I said I was the only person available (this wasn't true) but that I could only help them if they were prepared to accept me as I was. I did go on working with them for a while but when I mentioned this to my boss, she was furious and said that the council would always protect us against racism in clients.

Where there is a problem of this sort which cannot be resolved – and racial prejudice runs so deep in some people that this may well be the case – then refer the matter to your manager. Most employers have an active and helpful policy on such matters.

Summary

In this chapter we have looked at some of the basic principles of caring: encouraging independence in clients; how to weigh the balance of risks; encouraging the self-esteem that is so often damaged by being dependent on others for care; and protecting privacy. We have seen that preserving confidentiality is also important, as carers will inadvertently learn a lot about the private lives of clients; it is necessary to be clear as to who, if anyone, should be given confidential information. Finally, we have looked at the need to respect individuality as it may show in a client's culture, race, language or sexual preferences.

4

Helping with daily living

Almost all clients would prefer not to have to have your help with the most basic and personal tasks of daily living – eating, dressing, grooming, washing and going to the lavatory (usually described as 'toileting'). This chapter is about how to help clients with these jobs so that they preserve their dignity, independence and self-esteem in the difficult circumstances of being dependent on your care.

Eating

Virtually all carers have some responsibility for helping clients with eating and drinking. This may range from cooking and serving every meal to making and sharing the occasional cup of tea. As with so much work in caring, your role is much more important than it may at first appear.

There is more and more evidence to show that the poor quality and quantity of their food is unfortunately a prime cause of illness and death in vulnerable people in care. For instance, two hundred mentally handicapped patients in a Scottish hospital were said by one of their consultants to be seriously undernourished. They were eating far too little, not far short of half their recommended calorie intake. A further 600 patients were also underweight and their health was at risk as a result. A small number of patients at the same hospital had earlier been found to be dehydrated and had been referred to another hospital (*The Independent*, 7 December 1989). Why does this happen? There can be many causes and sometimes several of them could be at work at once:

- Dental disease affecting teeth and gums may mean that teeth have been extracted and that dentures no longer fit. Without teeth, chewing becomes impossible, and the range of acceptable foods will decrease. A bland soft diet may lead to constipation which in its turn decreases appetite.

- Appetite depends to some extent on a good sense of smell; this may have been lost in some clients, particularly the elderly.
- Other physical causes can include changes in the digestive system; for instance, older people may produce less saliva and without saliva food becomes unattractive to eat and difficult to swallow.
- Prescribed drugs may affect the way the body absorbs food.
- Eating alone is a necessity for many clients, yet eating is a social activity. Have you noticed, for instance, that you probably tend to eat a much larger meal when you are with other people than you do when you are alone? Many people who live alone find eating a chore to be got through rather than a ritual to be enjoyed.
- Some clients may not know how to cook, yet their circumstances force them to fend for themselves. A good example would be those widowers whose wives always did all the cooking and who now have little idea how to cope with preparing food from scratch, so rely on a monotonous diet of packets and tins.
- Some clients may be too poor to buy good food or too disabled to travel to find it.
- In institutional settings such as hospitals and nursing homes, the food may be so monotonous, of such poor quality and so unattractively presented that clients refuse it.
- Clients may have fixed ideas about nutrition, ideas formed many years previously, based perhaps on a time when their families were very poor. Such clients may find 'modern' or standard British food unacceptable.
- Where a client has become dependent on alcohol, his or her appetite will usually diminish. The alcohol also destroys the body's ability to absorb certain minerals and vitamins.

All these causes, especially if several combine, as they often do, may mean that clients eat and drink far too little. This in turn means that their general health will suffer. As a carer there is probably a limit to what you can do to change the buying and cooking practices of a large employer, and there is nothing you can do about physical changes associated with poor teeth, illness or old age. On several of the other factors, though, you could have a considerable impact.

Some clients will straightforwardly need help with the mechanics of eating. People with illnesses such as Parkinson's disease, arthritis, or multiple sclerosis may have difficulty holding conventional knives, forks and spoons, but there are many ingeniously adapted pieces of cutlery which can help; make sure your clients have the choice of using them if they want to, but remember it is the client's choice:

> Greg is a paraplegic eighteen-year-old with a little movement remaining in his arms. He had a motorbike accident eight weeks ago. I have offered him special cutlery and also a drinking cup because it would be easier for him to grip, but he refuses point blank. He says he won't use 'baby stuff'. As a result I watch his food get cold and him getting frustrated, but it's a sign of not 'giving in' to him, so that's what he must do.

> Arthur is a bedfast client who is slowly and gently dying. He was so pleased to be offered a special drinking cup after weeks of struggling with ordinary ones. He said it made everything less hassle.

Very ill or disabled clients may need to be fed because they can no longer hold even a spoon. This potentially humiliating experience can be made easier for clients by asking the client how he or she would like the feeding to be done, and by treating the matter cheerfully. Propping the client up securely, and covering neck and shoulders will prevent spilled food staining clothing. Do not overload the fork or spoon; that way more of it has a chance of reaching its destination securely.

Less ill or handicapped clients may still be missing out on their food intake because of simple things like where their food is placed. One study of a hospital ward showed what a large percentage of food remained uneaten because it was placed on a tray at the end of the patient's bed, and the patient was not well enough to make the effort to reach for it. So when you have to bring food to frail clients in bed, help them to sit up and put the food within very easy reach.

There are other ways in which you can try to encourage clients to increase the amount they eat. Ask what food they like and do everything you can to help them obtain it:

> The choice on our menu tended to be things like *either* 'sweet and sour' *or* curry. That is hopeless for elderly clients, so we

persuaded the kitchen that they ought to have a conventional English dish as well.

A lot of the clients only like sandwiches for tea and they'd be happy with things like fish paste or sandwich spread, anything that was soft. We still do sandwiches, but we use lots of different, nutritious soft fillings now.

Talking with them, laughing, joking and encouraging them to eat, showing an interest, that's all it needs.

In some situations, your employer may be open to suggestions for improving the variety of menus or the way the food is presented. It is often said that 'we eat with our eyes', meaning that food has to look as well as smell and taste appetizing. Contrasting the colour and texture and arranging the food prettily will often tempt a sluggish eater; exactly the same food might be left uneaten if it were just slapped on the plate.

Some residential homes and day centres have had much success in reviving flagging interest in food among clients by arranging 'Caribbean evenings' (or Indian, Chinese, or Italian evenings) where both food and entertainment are from that region. This creates a sense of fun, unpredictability and drama around food, making eating once more into an interesting process rather than a dreary chore.

You should also take every opportunity to encourage clients to eat with others rather than alone. In a residential home, eating is more enjoyable and more like a normal social activity if staff and clients eat together. In a hospital setting, encourage clients to join others at a central table rather than eating alone at their bedside. If you are a home care assistant, perhaps you could sit at a client's table sharing a cup of coffee while the client finishes her meal, or encourage her to take at least some of her meals with neighbours, family or other clients at a day centre. Clients who regularly and frequently eat with other people are more likely to keep up their food intake than clients who always eat alone.

You may be in a position directly to influence the buying and cooking of your client's food. If so, you have to try to balance two things: modern nutritional thinking and the preferences and choices of your client. The rules of healthy eating are simple: the emphasis is on plenty of 'unrefined' carbohydrates, that is, food such as potatoes, bread, rice, beans and pasta, which are high-energy foods, accompanied by lightly-cooked or raw fresh fruit and vegetables; fat should be eaten very moderately indeed, with sugar and salt reduced to a bare minimum.

This pattern of eating may be different from your client's own choices. It is not at all appropriate to try to force new ways of buying and cooking on clients. For most of us, food is an important part of our culture; it represents more than mere energy intake. Think, for instance, of the importance most people still attach to a Sunday roast or the Christmas turkey. Suggesting giving up such traditional feasts would bring howls of protest. None the less, there may be ways of suggesting improvements to a client's diet without appearing a know-all, patronizing, insensitive or unrealistic. Here are some ideas from carers who feel they have succeeded:

> I was working for three weeks with a very hard-up family where the father was in hospital and the mother was disabled. They seemed to live on a diet of chips, white bread and baked beans. I suggested cooked things like baked potato with grated cheese fillings, potato pies, cheap fish like coley (I cooked it with chips!) and added cheap fresh fruit from the market like bananas and tangerines. It was only a small set of changes, but it seemed to work; the kids liked it, anyway.

> Mr X had been widowed for the second time. He had no idea about cooking and was working his way through literally hundreds of tins he and his wife had accumulated in an enormous pantry. He developed scurvy because he was so short of vitamin C. Fortunately he had the sense to go to his doctor and she and the health visitor were a great help. Even so, part of my job was to show him how easy it was to cook cabbage, potatoes and other fresh vegetables or to grill a chop and a tomato. He learnt a few very basic dishes, but it made all the difference to his health.

> I show clients how easy it is to make soup from first-class ingredients, it's so simple to make and you can eat it without teeth.

Finally, you are likely to be in an excellent position to monitor how much and what clients actually eat and drink. Has Mr A left most of his food for the third or fourth day in succession? Has Mrs B complained that she cannot eat the toast at breakfast because her mouth ulcers are so bad? Has Miss C now been leaving out her

dentures for so long that her gums have shrunk and as a result she
constantly avoids food that needs to be chewed? Has anyone else
noticed that Mr D has not even lifted the lid on the plate delivered
to his bedside? All these are signs that clients could be at risk from
undernutrition.

   Various pieces of research* have identified common risk factors.
The main ones you should look out for are:

• fewer than eight main meals a week
• long gaps between meals (for example, 'supper' at 5.00 p.m. then
  nothing till breakfast at 8 a.m. the next day)
• minimal consumption of milk
• minimal consumption of fresh fruit and vegetables.
• a lot of food wasted
• loneliness and isolation
• difficulties with shopping
• physical or mental disability
• dependence on alcohol.

Where any of your clients fall into several of these categories, you
should look out for the classic signs of undernutrition: unusual weight
loss (and sometimes the rapid weight gain caused by eating a diet
high in fat and sugar) and lethargy. Talk to the client and try to find
out the reasons and alert your manager straight away if the problem
is not one that you can deal with on your own.

Dressing

There was a time not so long ago when it was quite usual for everyone
in a care institution to be given the same clothes. Perhaps it is
significant here to remember that part of the shame and humiliation of being in prison is that male prisoners have to wear a uniform
all the time. Those days are gone in residential care, but you may
still find yourself having to resist the temptation to control clients'
choices, and the whole process of helping them dress.

   First, never forget that exposing your body to others is normally
considered immodest, so help clients protect their modesty by
keeping their bodies covered as far as possible – for instance, by
covering themselves with a dressing gown.

*For instance L. Davies, *Three Score Years–And Then?* London, Heinemann
Medical Books.

Always ask what clothes the client would like to choose that day. Confused clients may forget that they have already worn a garment, or that the weather is warm, so a loose cotton shirt might be more comfortable than a tight, woollen one. In this case, pick up two cotton shirts or ask which the client would prefer. Choice is equally important when it comes to helping clients into their clothes. Does the client prefer to pull a jumper over her head, or does she like to put her arms in first? Asking will make it more likely that you will increase her feeling that she is not completely dependent on you.

It is also worth remembering that being dressed by someone else is potentially an uncomfortable physical experience. Most of us can still remember how it felt to be dressed by a parent who was in a hurry to get the task done: arms jerked up or down, ears pulled and the general feeling of being pushed and pummelled. Taking your time and letting the client do as much as possible for herself solves most of this problem, even if it takes longer. When dressing is complete, never miss an opportunity to compliment clients on their appearance, as long as you can do it without seeming patronizing or insincere.

Grooming

The same principles of choice, physical care and patience apply to hair care, nail care and shaving.

Hair

Hair care is perhaps particularly important. This care assistant in a nursing home comments on the difference that the hairdresser's visit can make to her clients:

> Even some of our frailest people will perk up and take more interest in life when the hairdresser visits. Someone whose hair has looked a bit straggly will suddenly seem a lot brighter when she's had a perm; having nice hair is such a basic part of feeling and looking good.

Equally, it can be distressing to clients who have always taken pride in their hair, if infirmity forces them to neglect it, as this home care assistant makes clear:

> I started visiting an elderly married couple because they were

both in poor health and had no one else who could do anything for them. One day the wife was in tears. She said she couldn't go out and she'd quarrelled with her husband. The reason was that she'd always taken particular care with her hair and now the arthritis in her shoulders meant that she couldn't do it and she couldn't afford a hairdresser. She showed me a picture of what it had been like; a really elaborate sort of sixties beehive with coil upon coil of hair. I offered to help. It was thick black hair and easy to arrange really, I remembered my mother having a similar style, it just needed time and dozens of hair pins. She was overjoyed. I don't suppose I'd done it as well as she did, but it was acceptable. The difference in her was astounding. It was a big step in restoring her confidence.

One danger is that carers can sometimes take too much interest in their clients' hair, trying to persuade them to adopt a hair style that clients feel is 'too young' or 'wrong' because it is not their choice. This woman, living in a sheltered housing scheme, recognized this kind of intervention as well meant, but highly irritating:

We had one warden who was a very nice person, a jolly, bouncing kind of young woman, but she did have this mission to turn us all into people with fashionable clothes and hair. When my heart condition meant that I'd got to the point where I couldn't go out to my own hairdresser, I had to use the one who comes here. Do you know, the warden would actually escort her into my flat and had the cheek to try to discuss with her how my hair should look. I know she meant well, but I've been doing my own hair and making my own decisions about it for wellnigh sixty-five years, so I certainly don't need any help and advice from her. She kept talking about how nice it would be for me to have something she called a 'feather cut'. I've no idea what that was, but I told her firmly that I didn't need her help. She actually looked quite offended!

It is nearly always a bad idea for carers to cut a client's hair. Hairdressing is a professional skill, so leave it to the professionals to carry it out.

Just as it is easy to cause clients discomfort when you help them with dressing, so it is equally easy to hurt people when you have to dress their hair, for instance by pulling too hard or being clumsy with elastic bands and grips. Asking the client for feedback on how you are doing is the best way to learn how to be efficient but gentle.

If you notice any disorders of the scalp or hair, it is important to let your manager know immediately. Most hair and scalp problems are not serious and can be readily treated; for instance, headlice can be effectively banished with a special shampoo and lotion but can cause more serious problems if they are ignored, as well as being potentially a widespread nuisance because they can infect a lot of scalps quickly in communities where people live closely together.

Multi-cultural issues are also important in hair care. If you are white, don't assume that the styles, methods, hair products, combs and brushes with which you are familiar will automatically be acceptable to black or Asian clients.

Nails

Nail care is usually more straightforward. More clients will be able to cut their own fingernails than can manage their toenails. Use clippers or scissors specially designed for the job and cut nails straight across; digging into the corners can cause painful infections. Some elderly people develop tough, thickened toenails; in such cases it helps to soak the feet first in warm soapy water and then dry them before cutting the nails. This process softens the nail and makes it much easier to cut. Do not attempt to deal with large corns and bunions; leave those to a chiropodist.

Shaving

Most male clients will be happy to continue to shave themselves because shaving can be carried out sitting down and in comfort. Allowing someone else to shave them often causes anxiety because clients may fear that you might cause small nicks and cuts. The secret of not doing so is, again, to be guided by the client and to take your time. Do not impose an electric shaver on someone who has always used a wet razor; most men have strong preferences for one or the other. Furthermore, a sudden change can cause skin irritations.

Hygiene is important because even skilful shaving can cause cuts. Where you have more than one client to shave, everyone should have their own equipment. Many infections are blood-borne; this includes serious viruses such as AIDS and hepatitis as well as much more trivial illnesses. Used razors must be safely disposed of in a 'sharps' box.

You may find that some women clients want help with shaving or with a depilatory cream to remove either underarm or facial hair. If so, it is vital to treat the matter sensitively and to handle the process in privacy and to keep the whole topic confidential. Facial hair, particularly, is likely to be a deeply embarrassing topic to the client.

Hygiene

Mouth care

Like shaving, mouth care is a routine that most clients will be able to handle perfectly adequately themselves. When you do feel you have to help, the first question to ask is, are you sure that you must? Having someone else clean your teeth is a serious surrendering of independence: if clients can carry on themselves, you should do all you can to encourage it. Sometimes there is a different problem: clients simply forget to clean their teeth. In these cases, try to re-establish this part of their routine, but let them actually carry it out themselves if they possibly can.

Where clients cannot clean their own teeth, ask how they like to have this task performed. Again, it is easy to be clumsy, so take it gently until you learn how to combine that client's wishes with a good standard of oral care. Use a soft bristle brush and be careful to clean all the teeth thoroughly – front, back and the biting surfaces. The main brushing motion should be from gums to biting surfaces. Dental floss and medicated wooden toothpicks are essential for removing the food debris between teeth that is the main cause of gum and tooth problems in adults.

Dentures should be handled carefully and cleaned thoroughly. Ask which method of cleaning and which product the client prefers. This will probably be dictated by the materials from which the dentures are made as different materials need to be cleaned and handled in different ways. Encourage clients to keep wearing their dentures as this will enhance self-esteem and increase the likelihood of the dentures remaining a good fit.

Like razors, toothbrushes should never be shared because of the risk of infection. Report any soreness, toothache, discoloration or lumps that you notice or that clients bring to your attention. Prompt dental care will normally prevent any problems becoming more serious.

Washing

Washing can sometimes be a source of difficulty with clients. Some clients may have got into the way of not washing and bathing frequently enough to prevent body odour becoming a problem. This can present taxing problems which test your ingenuity, tact and judgement. Here are some typical problems:

Mrs Bowness lives alone. She has rheumatoid arthritis and is visited by a home care assistant once a week. Whereas previously Mrs Bowness always looked scrupulously neat and clean, her clothes now look soiled and she smells strongly of body odour. Her son has contacted the home care assistant asking her to raise the problem with his mother. He says that her grandchildren are now refusing to visit her because they say 'Granny's so smelly'.

Mr Jenkins is a newcomer to a day-care centre. He has been a patient for 20 years in a hospital which is now closing. Other clients avoid sitting next to him at meals because, they say, he smells unpleasant. One other client has told him bluntly that he ought to wash. This has upset Mr Jenkins who is now refusing to go to the centre.

You will not need reminding of how sensitive a topic personal hygiene is. To be told that you smell unpleasant is a profoundly humiliating experience because it brings back memories of childhood dependence. It suggests sloppiness, dirtiness and letting important standards slip. It is not surprising, then, that other clients and colleagues will fight shy of telling the offender. How should you deal with such a problem?

Only you can judge what is right for your client in the particular situation you confront at the time, but some general rules may help. First, establish the facts. Is it actually true that a client smells unpleasant? If so, is it a constant problem or one that comes and goes?

Second, try to find out the cause. Reasons for developing a persistent body odour can range from a client's over-familiarity with his or her own smell, to loss of the sense of smell, physical difficulty with washing both themselves and their clothing, forgetting how to wash, incontinence or some physical disorder. You may be able to find the cause without confronting the client direct. For instance, you could ask whether the routines of daily living, including washing, are becoming more difficult. Your own observation may be enough to establish the cause. For instance, if you can see that Mrs Bowness's house is becoming dilapidated and cold, this may be enough to suggest that washing herself and her clothing is simply too much for someone with rheumatoid arthritis. You could offer help without suggesting that body odour is the problem. In the case of clients like Mr Jenkins, gentle questioning may reveal that in the hospital his bathing was organized for him; now that he is responsible for himself he straightforwardly forgets.

In some cases there is nothing for it but to tell the client gently that other people including yourself find it a problem. Say it straightforwardly but always give the client the chance to explain. Perhaps, again, there is some simple reason like not knowing how to use a washing machine, a broken washer on a hot tap or lack of opportunity to shop for deodorant and soap. Once the client has accepted the problem, then you should jointly work out a solution which gives the main responsibility to the client wherever possible. It would be pointless, for instance, for Mr Jenkins's carers to start organizing a formal bath time for him, since the whole point of his attending the day centre is to help him learn to look after himself. Instead, he could be encouraged to remind himself, by some method of his choice, of a suitable bathing routine.

Once you have agreed the solution, you will also need to keep an eye on how it works out in practice. Now that you have arranged laundry facilities for Mrs Bowness, has the problem disappeared? Has Mr Jenkins actually remembered to take baths?

The key to solving these problems successfully is to remember that you are negotiating with a fellow adult whose dignity is probably already fragile. Being straightforward, being gentle, being respectful and not imposing your solutions are all essential if there is to be a permanent solution that is acceptable to everyone.

You may have to help some clients actively, or even to wash them completely. For people who are still reasonably mobile, it may be enough just to make sure that they have everything they need: non-slip mat, towels, soap, flannels and clean clothes to hand. Test the temperature of the water: a tepid-to-warm temperature is better than the shock of water that is too cool or the risk of scalding from water that is too hot. Test the water with your elbow rather than your hand, as hands can withstand greater extremes of heat and cold than the rest of our bodies and will give a less reliable guide to temperature than an elbow.

Be sensitive to the need for privacy: close shower curtains, draw bed curtains and close doors, remaining within earshot if you have any doubts about a client's safety. For bedfast clients, keep as much of the body covered as you can, washing one section at a time. Even bedfast clients may actually be quite capable of doing the actual washing themselves. If they can, your role will simply be to hand them what they need.

When a male client has to be washed by a female carer there can be additional complications. For a start, both parties may feel self-conscious because of the sexual overtones that nakedness may have for one or both of them. The male client may, to his embarrassment, have an erection. If this happens you should remain calm and matter-of-fact. Do not show shock or disapproval or indeed read too much into the incident.

Simple rules of hygiene will help prevent the spread of infection. Every client should have two flannels, one for the face and one for the rest of the body. The flannels should be boiled frequently, and never shared between clients. Rinsing will remove residual soap from skin, while thorough 'blotting' dry with a soft towel will prevent chapping. In a care home or hospital, washing bowls should never be stacked one inside the other, but rinsed thoroughly and stored separately.

As with shaving, mouth and foot care, you should report anything unusual you notice in a client; especially bruises, lumps and swellings.

Toileting

Helping clients use a lavatory, commode or bedpan often causes anxiety both to carer and client. From babyhood we learn that our waste products, urine and faeces, are 'dirty' and that disposing of them is private and personal. Even a five-year-old will firmly close the lavatory door, leaving her mother outside. Being dependent on another person for help in this most personal of tasks can be intensely upsetting, as these clients describe:

> For the first four days that I needed to use a bedpan I was totally constipated, in spite of the kindness and tact of the auxiliary who brought it to me. I just couldn't open my bowels when I knew that I needed someone else to wipe my bottom for me. In the end I had to have an enema and that cured me in every way!

> Helpless . . . felt like a baby again . . . very aware of the horrible smell in the room and stains on the sheets, felt very ashamed.

> They left me sitting on the commode with my nightie round my waist for fifteen minutes. It was awful.

> What I find so difficult is having to ask for help. You're dependent on someone else in an aspect of your life where you've always been totally independent. If the staff are a bit slow responding, it makes me hopping mad.

For carers, too, this aspect of giving care can be trying:

> You feel embarrassed because they are embarrassed. You feel you're intruding, stepping into a part of their lives where you have no business to be.

> I couldn't help it, the first few times I had to help a client use the commode and had to wipe her bottom for her, I felt a dreadful wave of nausea and revulsion. I hope she didn't see it.

How can this aspect of the work be made easier for both sides? The same principles of choice should apply to toileting as to every other aspect of care work. When a client has a strong preference to go on using the lavatory, then your job will be to try everything in your power to help her do so, even if it takes you longer than it would to put a commode in her room. Going on using the normal facilities for as long as possible is clearly the ideal for the client. Quite often it is only the physical difficulties of making the journey which stand in the way; adding aids like grab rails and ramps or providing a human assistant may be all that is required. This home care assistant describes how she helped her client solve this problem:

> Mrs Samuels is determined to go on living at home as long as possible, but the loo arrangements were causing a problem.

The only decent one was upstairs, near her bedroom, but she hated being confined to her bedroom because she said it made her feel like an invalid. With the Council's help, we all worked out a scheme whereby the old outside loo was 'brought indoors' by knocking down a wall, a radiator and a shower were installed there and we turned her large parlour downstairs into a bed-sitting room. She holds court there now with streams of visitors all day long. Putting a rail at key places between her room and the shower room means she's quite happy that she can manage. It's made a tremendous difference to her confidence.

Sometimes, it is not so much the journey that is difficult, as the problems the client has in sitting down and getting up from the lavatory itself. This is an easier issue to resolve. A whole range of simple gadgets and aids can transform the problem; for instance, an extension to the lavatory seat which raises it substantially, makes sitting down and getting up much easier; tip-up seats can help disabled people with the getting-up part of the process, toilet tongs can help clients continue to wipe their own bottoms rather than depending on your help. Your employer will have a list of such aids and you should not hesitate to ask for access to it when you can see that a particular aid will help a client.

Occasionally, clients are discouraged from independent use of the lavatory because of fears for their safety. Only you, the client and your manager can assess each individual case, but it is probably always worth asking whether the risks could be made smaller, with some help. If the client is subject to blackouts, could you wait outside the lavatory with the door half open? If the client is subject to falls, have risks from slippery floors been eliminated, for instance by making sure that floors are carpeted or that there are non-slip mats in place? Is the lavatory itself in impeccable working order so that there is no risk of the client slipping and falling while struggling with the flush?

For clients who do need your help, your own attitude is one of the keys to helping them overcome any embarrassment or humiliation they may feel. Remaining friendly, unembarrassed and matter-of-fact yourself will help you both:

> I go to great pains to avoid baby-talk and a patronizing attitude. I sometimes hear other care assistants saying things like 'now, so and so, time for a wee-wee' and it makes me cringe.

Asking yourself how you would like to be treated in their place is the way to get it right. Never ask people when others can overhear you, always maintain people's dignity.

This last point is important. Maintaining privacy is absolutely essential. Where clients have to use a commode in a bedroom, leave them to it and close the door or curtains wherever possible. When you leave the room, knock and wait for a reply before coming back in. If you leave the room, do not forget the client; nothing can be worse than being left propped on a bedpan or commode and being utterly helpless to leave it until your carer returns. Where clients need to be reminded about going to the lavatory, give them the reminder privately.

Using a bedpan or bottle can be uncomfortable for clients. Remembering to warm the bottle or bedpan with warm water and then drying it can solve this problem. Sprinkling talcum powder on a bedpan can also help prevent skin sticking uncomfortably. Turning the bedclothes back without exposing the clients' body helps preserve privacy and dignity.

Hygiene is important, especially when commodes, bedpans and bottles are involved. Remove any soiled clothing or bedding immediately. Keep the equipment scrupulously clean by washing, rinsing with disinfectant and then drying. Wash your own hands thoroughly and make sure clients do so, too. There are now many excellent air-fresheners which will help disguise unpleasant smells, and it will always help to air a room thoroughly by opening windows and doors, but beware of sudden changes of temperatures and draughts in cold weather.

Bowels and bladder are excellent indicators of general health, so you should look out for any changes or abnormalities which might indicate problems. In particular, be alert to changes in quantity, colour, consistency or smell. Blood in urine or faeces should also always be taken seriously, as should any client reporting pain in passing urine or faeces.

Incontinence

If toileting demands skill and patience, then dealing with incontinence does even more so. Incontinence means that voluntary control of bowels and bladder has been lost, so that the client is subject to humiliating 'accidents'. The dreadful embarrassment and shame of such events can seem unbearable, as these clients report:

> It began as 'dribbling' when I coughed or sneezed, but after a bit it began to happen when I did something as minor as just walking down my front steps. I had to start wearing a sanitary towel, but that rubbed and was very uncomfortable. Fortunately I had the sense to mention it to my health visitor and she got me medical treatment. Otherwise I'd have ended up avoiding everyone and feeling like a leper.

> You spend your whole time worrying about where the lavatory is and whether you're going to get there in time or not. I often don't, so there's the whole horrible business of stains on your clothing which means that other people have to know.

Causes

Urinary incontinence is more common than faecal incontinence. Its causes include muscle weakness (as in 'stress incontinence' on sneezing or laughing), bladder infections, damage to the central nervous system as a result of a stroke or tumour, drugs prescribed for high blood pressure which affect all the muscles, including those around the bladder, senile dementia, drugs prescribed to get rid of excess fluid, physical handicap, prostate gland problems in men, and simple inability to reach the lavatory and unfasten clothes quickly.

Faecal incontinence can be caused by strokes, senile dementia, a type of constipation called 'impacted faeces' which also induces an overflow of faeces. Inability to reach the lavatory in time may also be a cause.

You will hear some carers claim that there is another type of incontinence, described as 'wilful incontinence' – that is, people who are incontinent on purpose. The theory goes that such people use incontinence as a way of trying to punish their carers and to draw attention to themselves.

Treatment

Much incontinence is curable, so it is a great mistake as a carer to

imagine that incontinence is 'inevitable' or 'normal'. It is not inevitable and is always abnormal, so the first step with any client suffering
from incontinence is to make sure that he or she has immediate access
to medical help. If the cause is a bladder infection, then antibiotics
will usually bring about a cure; surgery may be able to correct
problems caused by physical blockage such as a tumour or an enlarged
prostate gland. Where faecal impaction is causing faecal incontinence
the cure is often simple – a radical change in diet – as this residential
home proprietor describes:

> I bought my first care home some years ago as a going concern.
> The first thing I discovered was that virtually every resident
> was seriously constipated and that several were incontinent
> as a result. The misery this created was enormous. Virtually
> every resident was using laxatives! The cause wasn't hard to
> find; a dreadful diet of white bread, cake, sugar, biscuits, no
> fresh vegetables and fruit to speak of. I immediately introduced
> alternatives: soft wholemeal bread, bran muffins, brown rice,
> whole cereals like 'Shredded Wheat', salads, unpeeled fruit,
> plenty of fluids, all presented in ways that were easy for elderly
> people to eat (for instance, the oranges were peeled and
> presented in segments, the salads always chopped in small
> pieces). Within about ten days there was nobody on laxatives
> and no one with faecal incontinence.

Where the problem is damaged muscle control, the solution is to
encourage clients to make regular and frequent use of the lavatory,
commode or bedpan. Every two hours is usually considered about
right. Physiotherapy can also help strengthen muscles and most
physiotherapists can teach all but very confused clients how to carry
out a programme of exercises that will strengthen the muscles around
the anus and bladder.

So-called 'wilful incontinence' is in a different category. Some carers
deny that it exists, and say that it is a hurtful label invented by people
who cannot see that clients would always and in every circumstance
prefer continence to incontinence. Others claim that deliberate incontinence is an effective way for clients to make a protest. If this is so,
then you certainly have to take it seriously, since a client's unhappiness and discontent would have to be extraordinarily major for such
a high price to be paid in the shame and discomfort that ensue.

If you suspect wilful incontinence in a client, then the only solution is to discover what lies behind the behaviour. You have to assume that the client is unhappy, but what is the cause? Perhaps it is significant here that 'wilful incontinence' is not something that most home care assistants will ever describe. If it exists, it seems to be a condition that institutions create, so the solution will be in altering the way the institution treats the client.

However, some carers have had success with confused clients whom they suspect of deliberate incontinence by using a tactic designed to reward the approved behaviour (remaining dry) and discourage the disapproved behaviour (wetting). This system is based on the assumption that deliberate incontinence is designed to attract attention. So a wet client will be changed with minimum fuss and attention in a straightforward, matter-of-fact way. A client who is checked and found to be dry, on the other hand, will be rewarded with praise, encouragement or even with a token that can be exchanged for sweets.

However, we have to suspect that an even better and less patronizing tactic might be simply to increase the total amount of attention that staff give to clients and to create a stimulating and interesting environment in which clients do not feel driven to the desperate lengths of wetting themselves in order to attract five minutes of their carers' time.

Where the cause of incontinence is inability to get to the lavatory quickly, the solution is twofold. First, do everything you can to keep clients mobile. The more clients keep themselves physically fit with gentle exercise, the more likely they are to be able to reach the lavatory in time. So encourage walking and gentle exercising of all sorts to keep muscles and the circulatory system in trim. Second, encourage regular and frequent trips to the lavatory so that bladder and bowels never need to be emptied in a hurry and make sure that clients can loosen clothes easily, perhaps using velcro fastenings instead of zips and buttons.

There may be aspects of the environment itself which can help – for instance, making sure that the route to the lavatory is short, well lit at all times and, in institutions, clearly signposted in large, conspicuous letters. Doors should be easy to open and lavatories themselves large enough to allow for manoeuvring walking aids. The room should be well heated and well ventilated with a call button to give clients confidence that if they do get into difficulties, someone will come to help.

Nighttime incontinence has the same range of causes as daytime incontinence and you need to approach it in the same way. Additional preventive measures can include, avoiding giving sleeping pills whenever possible, because their use means that clients often sleep through the normal warning signals from the bladder; avoiding drinking a lot of fluid late at night; cutting down on drinks like tea, coffee and cocoa which contain caffeine and therefore can irritate the bladder. Other strategies include remembering to keep the room gently lit at night so that confused clients are not even more confused by waking up in darkness. A fairly low bed with a firm mattress, grab rails and supports to hand will also make it easier for clients to get out of bed unaided.

This care assistant describes the approach to nighttime incontinence at her place of work which successfully combines several of these tactics at once:

> I have done night duty for many years in a local nursing home. We have developed an approach to residents with enuresis (urinary incontinence while asleep) which has proved its worth. First of all, every room has nightlights. We are always sympathetic, always caring, but we work out a plan *with each client* for avoidance. This will vary from one to another, but a typical one would be to agree to cut down fluids after 6 p.m., to encourage the client to wake up in response to signals from the bladder (a lot of them describe *dreaming* that they need to go) and if they are really nervous about it, to agree to wake them at a particular time in the night so that they can empty their bladder.
>
> We also discourage the use of sleeping pills except where absolutely unavoidable because we were finding that the pills suppress the client's natural instinct to wake up when the bladder is full. We now only have real problems with people who have advanced dementia; none of these tactics is reliable with them.

This approach works for several reasons. First, and most importantly, it involves the client in thorough consultation and discussion, emphasizing the importance for clients of remaining independent and of taking as much responsibility for themselves as they can manage. Second, the problem is approached optimistically – the client is given hope that a solution can be found. Finally, several tactics are tried at once in a way that encourages flexibility and adaptability. This approach is usually described as 'promoting continence', emphasizing that continence is the norm and that it is a standard that can be aimed for and reached.

Where continence is impossible through mental or physical disability, then there is now a huge range of aids that can help the client attain 'social continence', that is, the state where clients continue to be incontinent, but it is no longer an embarrassment to them or others. These aids will vary from catheters (a hollow tube attached to the bladder at one end and a collection pouch at the other) to dribble pouches for men and incontinence pads of different sorts, including the type that allows moisture to pass through so that the wearer remains reasonably dry.

Soiled incontinence pads should be disposed of carefully in sealed bags and linen that has been soiled with faeces or urine put in a separate sealed bag for specialist laundering which will reduce the risk of contamination and infection. As with any aspect of toileting, pay careful attention to your own and your clients' hygiene by scrupulous washing including nails. You may need to use barrier creams on clients who suffer from urinary incontinence, otherwise sores and rashes can add to the client's problems.

You will also need to give some thought to clothing for incontinent clients. Fabric which is easily washable, colour-fast, creaseproof and fast-drying is best. The clothes themselves need to be easily opened but also to be secure once fastened. Shoes and slippers will often encounter puddles, so waterproof footwear and washable slippers are essential. Specialist organizations such as the Disabled Living Foundation can advise on the ingenious ways in which 'normal' clothing can be adapted so that the client does not feel or look conspicuous. One other point here: never leave unused incontinence pads on view where visitors or other clients can see them. Keep them stored discreetly out of sight.

Probably the most important aspect of the whole task is your own stance. Tact, patience and understanding are the only possible attitudes. Showing any revulsion or nausea will make an already vulnerable client feel a lot worse. How do experienced carers cope with this aspect?

At first I was really worried about doing what carers called 'the dirty round', dealing with the three or four residents who always fouled their beds. The first time I nearly gave up there and then, but I came to see that the poor old things just couldn't help it, and it was our job to make sure we helped them keep whatever shreds of dignity remained. I told myself it was part of the job and now I'm proud to be able to do it without flinching.

Originally I wondered how I'd cope as I'd found even my own children's nappies revolting and an adult bowel produces so much more than a baby's! But it soon got to be an everyday routine, and the new system we have here of checking the patients who are liable to involuntary voiding means that we can often prevent it. Many of them have regular patterns, so if we get them on to the commode, they often oblige and that's so much easier for them and us.

They can't help it and they need someone to do it, it's just part of the work. I try to do it as caringly and tenderly as everything else, it's no different really.

Reducing the risks of infection

In helping clients with so many of the tasks of daily living, it is essential to reduce the risks of infection as far as possible. This applies whether you work in a residential home, a hospital, or visit clients in their own homes.

Infections can be transferred in many ways: through fomites (substances which are able to absorb and transmit contagion on towels or clothing); through *breathing* infected air; by bacteria or viruses entering *broken skin*, for instance via a cut; or by *eating and drinking* infected food. By keeping to certain strict rules of hygiene, you can cut down the risks both to yourself and to your clients.

- Clean hands are the foundation of minimizing the spread of infection. The routine for thorough washing is to use special liquid soap supplied in a dispenser, to work up a thorough lather, pressing it hard into fingers and high up your wrists, to rinse and then to carry out the whole process again. Be careful to use lavish amounts of soap under your nails, cleaning them with a disposable stick if necessary. Dry your hands thoroughly, preferably with a dry air heater or on a disposable towel which is thrown away safely after use. A communal towel will harbour germs and should be avoided. If you are a home carer working with clients whose own standards of hygiene are poor, then take your own towel for your use.

You should wash your hands before and after: serving food; washing and dressing clients; handling dressings; taking clients to the lavatory; handling bedpans and commodes and fouled linen; and using the lavatory yourself. Keeping your nails short will reduce the surfaces on which dirt and bacteria can be trapped.

- Always wear overalls, and for dirty jobs, wear a disposable plastic apron over them. Use rubber or disposable plastic gloves wherever possible. When you have to carry soiled linen, hold it well away from you and change your apron afterwards. Dispose of used incontinence pads in sealed plastic bags. Most local authorities have a special collection service as it is normally considered wise to treat these waste materials as unsuitable for mixing with normal household waste.
- Clean up spills and stains immediately, especially from urine and faeces. Use a suitable proprietary detergent and then disinfectant to prevent bacteria and odours spreading.
- Encourage clients to develop the same exacting standards of hygiene themselves; especially in relation to the use of the lavatory.
- If you work in residential care, fight like a tiger against communal use of razors, toothbrushes, toothmugs, denture cups, flannels and towels. These avenues of infection should be closed off completely.
- Keep away from direct contact with clients if you have a boil, skin abrasion, a cold or sore throat.

Summary

This chapter has looked at some of the essential skills for helping clients with the tasks of daily living. It has explored how to help clients maintain an adequate diet, and how to encourage choice and self-esteem where dressing and grooming are concerned; it has suggested some tactics for dealing with clients who neglect washing themselves or their clothing. The section on toileting has emphasized the importance of preserving dignity and privacy as well as looking at some possible ways of promoting continence. Finally, some basic rules of hygiene have been suggested as essential ways of limiting the spread of infection.

5

Listening and talking

Why does communication matter?

This chapter is about how to communicate well with clients. It is highly likely that you have been drawn to caring as a job because you are already an excellent communicator. If so, this is a considerable plus because listening and talking competently are fundamental skills that you need to do the job well. When communication is good, it is easy to take it for granted. It is often only when it fails that you realize how critically important it can be:

> I know we aren't supposed to have favourites, but I can't help liking some clients more than others. One of my nicest clients recently got taken into hospital at very short notice and died before I had a chance to go and see her. It turned out that she had an advanced breast cancer. I feel dreadful about it now, because I realize that she'd been trying to raise the subject and ask my opinion about it for almost a year. Every time she'd said things like 'I suppose we're all likely to get cancer at some point if we live long enough', or 'Do you think it's worth going to the doctor for a check up at my age?', I'd assumed she just wanted general reassurance. I hadn't realized that this was a symptom of her worry and that I should have sat down with her and said 'Why do you ask?' or 'Tell me how you feel your own health is at the moment.' Instead, I just said cheerful things like 'Oh, you'll live to be a hundred – you needn't worry about that'. The awful thing was that I was literally the only person she saw where this kind of chat was possible.

This care assistant is being too hard on herself because, in the end, the client's health was the client's responsibility, not hers. However, she is right to be self-critical of her ability to listen out for more than is apparently being said: listening well is more than simply registering the words that are being spoken, just as talking well is more than merely speaking them.

Good communication is an important skill for carers. Here is an example of its successful use, described by a care assistant working in a residential home for elderly people:

> I always have good conversations with Sam because it takes ages to get him out of bed, toileted, shaved and dressed in the mornings. I gradually began to realize that he'd got it into his head that he was going to be thrown out of the home because he knew he was needing more and more care, and he knew the owners preferred able-bodied people. By encouraging him to tell me about it, I was able to get Mr —, the proprietor, to come and reassure him that there was absolutely no question of his being asked to leave. The difference in him was amazing. He was back to his old cheerful self in no time.

Real communication with clients is important as a way of their being able to alert you to physical or emotional problems. Confronting such problems early can often prevent them growing into major issues later.

But effective communication is also one of the rewards of the job for you. A warm, mutually satisfying relationship with clients is built on the foundation of good listening and talking.

We have already seen that this can be important as a way of anticipating and short-circuiting a client's problems. But it can also matter if you have to act confidently to represent clients' interests. This process is often described as 'advocacy', a term drawn from the legal profession where a lawyer is also an advocate for a client's. interests at law.

Suppose you see from your visits or from observation that a client is facing some kind of crisis. It may be a crisis about money, about health, or about the conditions in which he or she lives. You may need to take up your client's case with your own bosses or with colleagues from another department. You cannot do this with certainty or confidence unless you have a firm basis of communication with your client, as illustrated by this home care assistant:

> I became very concerned about Mrs Rampal because her council

flat was deteriorating to the point where it was affecting her health. My boss eventually took this up for me, but the Housing Department immediately came back at me saying that Mrs Rampal wasn't all that concerned and that she was on their repairs list but she was not a priority. I knew her well, because even though she doesn't speak good English she understands it OK and we'd got a really good relationship going. I knew I was on very firm ground about how she felt. With my help she eventually wrote several letters and we kept the pressure up. Within six weeks, the repairs were done! I couldn't have convinced them if I hadn't been able to give so much detail on how she felt, no matter what factual things I could have said about how the place looked.

You may also find yourself needing to give information and advice to clients. For instance, you may need to tell a client how to change a dressing, how to reheat food, how to change the bag on a vacuum cleaner or how to describe symptoms to their doctor. You cannot do this effectively unless there is trust between you, and trust is built on the foundations of effective communication.

What gets in the way of good communication?

Since it is so clear that first-rate communication is essential to the job of caring, why does it frequently go wrong? One of the main reasons is that good communication takes time. It is often easier to assume that you know what a client thinks because you are busy and have so many other clients to attend to. However, in the long run, cutting communication short and failing to create opportunities to listen may simply be storing up bigger problems for later on. For instance, in one home, the matron did not tell clients that a major piece of building work was going to start. Rumours swept the home, all of them inaccurate and exaggerated – for instance that fees were to be increased by 50 per cent. There was a good deal of unhappiness among the clients. One of the ways it surfaced was a marked increase in continence 'accidents' and in conflict between groups and individuals. This led to far more difficulties for the staff than if there had been a straightforward announcement followed by opportunities for people to express their worries.

Another frequent communication problem is that staff always keep control of all conversations. How often, for instance, do you find yourself choosing the topic, then both opening and closing the conversation with a client? If this is always the pattern, then it will be hard for clients to raise the matters that they want to discuss.

Another variant on this communication trap is to find yourself always addressing clients with questions that only need the answer 'yes' or 'no'. 'Are you all right, Mary?' 'Is your son coming to visit you today?' 'Do you want me to warm up this food for you?' 'Bowels OK, are they?'

In some situations, proper communication is made difficult simply because there is nowhere private to talk. One of the worst features of the old-fashioned long-stay hospital was the minute amount of private space allowed each patient. Even if it was possible to draw curtains around each bed, the chances were that several people could hear every word of the conversation – hardly the right atmosphere to encourage confidences. If you work in any kind of residential care you may find it takes effort to find privacy for a real conversation.

Even if you can find privacy, there may be problems created by difficulties of language and culture. When clients speak a different language and come from a different culture or have a different religion it may be much harder to communicate effectively with them:

> Many years ago I had to deliver meals on wheels to an Asian client. I knew that she didn't eat pork, but I couldn't understand why one day and for several days following, she waved my meals away. I thought she was implying that the food was awful or something. I feel very ashamed now that I had no idea about Ramadan. As a devout Muslim she was trying to tell me that she had to fast during the daytime!

As well as these high-profile difficulties over food there may also be less obvious difficulties over social customs. For instance, Chinese clients may find it hard to accept offers of help. It is polite in their culture to refuse help for at least the first few times it is offered, and there may also be 'loss of face' in having to accept financial or other help from the host society. Unless you are alert to these problems, they can create enormous barriers to successful communication.

There may also be problems associated with physical or mental disability which make communication difficult. A confused client, a client with a visual or hearing impairment, means that you have to be more than usually skilful and sensitive in your approach and will probably need specialist advice from voluntary and statutory organisations who deal with such clients all the time and understand their special needs.

The skill of empathy

To communicate successfully with clients, you need to be able to see the world from the client's perspective and to understand the difference between 'sympathy' and 'empathy'.

People outside caring may sometimes ask you how you can bear the emotional burden of working constantly with frail and vulnerable clients. They assume, perhaps, that because your work exposes you to other people's distress, you yourself are bound to become distressed because of the *sympathy* you want to show clients. Alternatively, you may find yourself being accused of 'becoming hard' precisely because you are able to deal with clients' distress without bursting into tears yourself.

The secret is that there is a correct balance between the two which is summed up by the word *empathy*. To communicate effectively with clients you need to be able to show empathy. This means listening carefully, showing that you are listening and understanding the problem but then helping the client find the solution that is right for him. *Sympathy*, on the other hand, means identifying with the client so strongly that you feel what he feels, you cry when he cries, feel worried when he feels worried, and so on.

An empathetic listener is more useful than a sympathetic one because the empathetic listener remains calm. She is on your side, but still able to help. The sympathetic listener is too emotional to be able to think and act logically. The sympathetic listener says: 'Oh, I do understand. If I were you I'd . . .' The empathetic listener says, 'Oh, I do understand. Of course I'm not you, and only you can decide what to do. Why don't we take a look at the problem together?'

How to communicate empathy

Many people are naturally good at communicating empathy. Most of us find that it is a skill that comes with increased awareness and practice because it has so many different aspects. Some of them are highlighted here.

Make sure that your 'body language' shows empathy

Communication is more than just listening and talking. We show
how we are feeling in a situation by facial expression, by how we
sit, stand and walk. When you are feeling tense, for instance, you
may sit shoulders hunched and with your legs tightly crossed or your
fists clenched. If a problem at work or at home makes you angry,
you may find yourself pushing your chair away from the table or
turning your body from the group as a way of showing that you do
not want to be associated with the opinions other people are
expressing. Another common way of showing disapproval or disagree-
ment is to cross your arms over your chest. This conveys the message:
'you needn't think any of your ideas are going to touch me!'

To show empathy with clients you need to use positive body
language (see Figure 2). Generally speaking, this will involve postures
such as standing close, but not too close, leaning forward and making
sure that you do not cross your arms. Keeping your palms up is
another 'open' or 'receptive' gesture.

Keep plenty of eye contact

When we are feeling angry and hostile, we tend to avoid direct eye

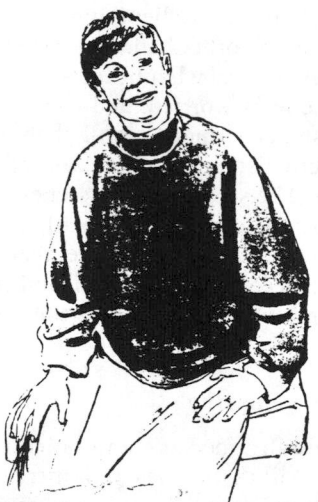

Figure 2 Positive body language

contact. Letting eye contact drift away also indicates boredom: you are bound to have had experience of how disconcerting it can be if you are talking to someone whose gaze suddenly shifts over your shoulder. So to demonstrate empathy you need to do the opposite: to make sure you look directly at clients, not so much that you unsettle them, but probably more than you would in an ordinary social conversation.

Stay on the same physical level

Never try to have a serious conversation with a client while you are standing up and she is sitting down. Always crouch at her level if she is already sitting down. Speaking from 'on high' suggest dominance. Your eyes need to be on the same level.

Do not be afraid of silence

Show by the relaxed way you are sitting and listening that silence is all right. A peaceful, reflective silence is often valuable and a good way for a client to collect thoughts. You can say 'Mmm' or 'Yes, I see' without adding any more yourself. This is a highly effective way of prompting people to speak because it gives 'permission' to talk at length. This is why a filmed interview will always include shots call 'noddies'. These simply consist of a couple of minutes of the interviewer nodding – seriously, laughingly, thoughtfully – all of which can be slotted in at points where the interview has been edited.

Use verbal prompts

These are those useful little phrases such as 'oh dear', 'golly', 'do go on', 'tell me more', 'what happened then?', 'oh, I see', which prompt the client to go on talking. Keeping looking alert and not too relaxed will convey interest in what the client is saying.

Keep observing the client

Just as you should keep monitoring your own behaviour, you should also keep a close eye on your client. Is she avoiding eye contact with you? Is she folding her arms or turning away from you? Is she raising or lowering her voice? If so, is it because of you and your body language, or is it because of the topic you are discussing?

Ask open-ended questions

These are questions that cannot be answered 'yes' or 'no'. They begin with phrases like 'Tell me', (a specially useful one) or 'How did you . . .', or 'Why was it that you . . .', or 'Can you describe how you felt when . . .' These phrases invite lengthy answers. They give the client permission to speak without interruption. They also give no clues about what your own opinion is. Thus they are the best kind of question to ask because you are trying to encourage the client to express her view, not to mimic yours.

Smile and look friendly

Here is another obvious way that we communicate without actually speaking. If you know that your normal facial expression is rather serious, make sure that in communicating with clients you cultivate a consciously friendly expression. A frowning face can unwittingly suggest that you are disapproving or hostile.

Keep your voice soft

A quiet, slow friendly tone communicates the idea that you can be trusted and that you have plenty of time.

Show that you are listening by reflecting back what the client is saying

This is an important aspect of empathy. What it means is that when a client is describing a difficult problem or struggling to express feelings on a topic that matters a great deal to him or her, you show how carefully you have listened by reflecting back what has been said.

Let us suppose that one of your clients in a residential home begins to talk to you about how much she dislikes eating with so many other people. She says: 'I'm not used to eating with all these people at the same time and place. I used to like eating what I wanted to eat when I liked and propping a book up in front of me. Here I feel

I can't. I've got to listen to all this silly chatter and conversation when I'd rather eat on my own.' The empathetic reply is to summarize or *reflect* what she has just said, by saying something like 'Mmm, yes, I see . . . you mean you'd prefer the freedom and privacy of being able to eat alone?' Try to avoid using the same words and always end on a question.

The value of this kind of response is, first, that it shows you have been listening hard. Second, it is a check on how accurately you have heard the client because if your summary is inaccurate, you have given her a change to correct it because you have phrased your comment as a question.

If your employer sends you on a training course, you may find that 'reflecting' is one of the first skills you are given the chance to practise. Usually it is done in pairs: each person takes it in turns to speak while their partner reflects back what they have said. When you have never done this before it can be surprisingly difficult; a sign perhaps of how rarely we actually give another person our full attention.

Giving advice

You may often find that you have to give advice to clients – for instance, about diet and cooking, safety in their homes or rooms, drugs and medicines, grants and benefits, using household or other equipment, and so on. These will tend to be topics where there is a recognized opinion on what it is sensible to do.

The temptation in such circumstances is to give clients a mini-lecture. You have the information and you dump it on the client. Unfortunately, this is not an effective way to communicate. It is often described as the 'hole-in-the-head theory' of giving people information – as if clients had a hole in their head through which advice and guidance could be poured:

> Our GP is a very nice woman, but when she tells you what's wrong with you and what tablets you have to take, she gabbles on and I can never follow her half the time. She knows I'm deaf because she got me my hearing aid, but she also seems to forget that one gets very nervous and frightened going to the doctor and that gets in the way of taking in what she says.

A better way of approaching this kind of situation is, again, to use

Caring for people

an empathetic approach. First, what does the client need to know or to do? Answering these questions will almost certainly mean that the client talks more than you do. Here is an example of successfully given advice, which shows how this approach works out in practice:

> I work with blind and partially sighted clients living in their own homes. One of my clients, Mr Jenkins, was given a microwave cooker by his daughter. It was a good present because it is so much safer than radiant heat. Obviously my client couldn't read the instruction book, so I went through it all very briefly and in a very non-specialist-cook way. I felt confident because I've been using a microwave myself for years. Then I got Mr Jenkins to go through the whole routine himself, very slowly, actually handling a dish with something in it, using the controls, checking that he was identifying the timing buttons correctly (he was). Then I got him to explain to me what the safety rules were and how he proposed to adapt them. I also asked him what food and dishes he thought he'd find it useful to try and got him to talk me through how he'd cook them. I suggested that on my next visit we discuss any of the practical problems there proved to have been. Altogether I'm sure I fulfilled my aim on these occasions, which is: client talks four times as much as I do!

Here the advice given is soundly based on good information, phrased in a way the client can understand, and closely linked to the client's own needs. The carer checked back on how well the client had understood and there was a mutually agreed plan for following it up.

A good information base

Always check the status of any information you are passing on to clients. Are you really sure that a Pyrex dish is safe in a microwave? If not, who can you go to in order to find out? Is it really the case that Neurofen (available as an over-the-counter drug) is the same as the Brufen recommended by your client's sister for the relief of arthritic pain? You may already know that, yes, Neurofen is part of the Brufen family, but you would be wise to encourage your client to consult her doctor to double-check. If you have any doubts about the information you give clients, then always take advice from someone who has specialist knowledge.

Agree the goals

In Mr Jenkins's case, the goal was clear: he needed to be able to use the microwave safely on his own to cook a number of simple dishes. A less skilled home carer might have tried to foist other goals on him – for instance, to understand the workings of the magnetron, or to be capable of cooking a six-course dinner for two. Both these goals would have been completely irrelevant to his needs. Establish at the start what goal the client would like to reach, discuss it, help modify it if necessary, but remember that ultimately it has to be the client's goal not yours, otherwise he or she is unlikely to be able to reach or stick to it.

Linking to the client's needs

When advice is offered, and rejected, the reason is nearly always the same: it was not perceived by the client as relevant. For instance, it is no use telling a family barely existing on a very small income that they should buy more fresh fruit and vegetables. Most likely they already know that. The problem is that they have far too little money left over from buying staple food like bread and potatoes to be able to afford the fresh produce. Telling people that they should give up smoking is also unlikely to be a new idea. Asking them what needs smoking meets and why it is so difficult to stop is far more likely to give you information which will help you phrase the advice in a way that can be linked to the client's underlying needs.

Use appropriate language

Skilful carers will always adapt what they say to the language the client herself uses and understands. Where clients do not speak English or are profoundly deaf you must find an interpreter; where clients are confused or suffering from mental handicap, you must stick to short simple words, repeating things as many times as seems necessary.

Never be tempted to use your professional jargon. What would most clients make, for instance, of some of the favourites from social work,

such as 'interaction' or 'intervention'? Most successful communication sticks to this simple rule: *Keep it short, keep it simple*.

   One famous example of the virtues of brevity is this:

The Lord's Prayer	54 words
The Ten Commandments	294 words
American Declaration of Independence	300 words
EEC Regulation on the exporting of duck eggs	269,111 words

Which of these do you think rate most highly as pieces of effective
communication?

Check for understanding

An uninterrupted flow of words is almost impossible to follow. Most
of us are lost after only a few sentences, especially if the whole subject
is unfamiliar and if we are tense or worried. Pause after a few
sentences and say 'What would you like to ask me about that?'; allow
a long enough pause for the client to raise anything she has not
understood.

   At regular points throughout the conversation you can also look
for ways to get the client to repeat the whole explanation or demonstration, or whatever it is, back to you. Beware of making it sound
like a test: you should suggest it as a way of helping her make sure
she understands, rather than appearing as if you are looking for ways
to catch her out.

Agree the next steps

There may not need to be any next steps; if not, that's fine, but usually
there will be. How are the drugs going? Is the use of the microwave
creating any problems? Has the housing benefit been paid? Always
agree with the client what should happen next and keep your half
of the bargain. You may, in addition, need to help the client find
more sources of advice, readjust her goals, or put her in touch with
other people.

Counselling and giving advice: the difference

For many of your clients, you may be one of the few other human beings they see regularly. This can sometimes mean that you feel especially responsible when they ask you for advice or expect you to be able to help them solve complicated problems. Here are some typical dilemmas reported by carers:

> Mr Wallace keeps falling down. He lives alone and I know that he dreads falling, perhaps over the weekend, and no one knowing. He's constantly asking me if I think he ought to try to move to sheltered housing or whether he's better off where he is. He loves his independence and I can't see him putting up with the limits on his freedom, but on the other hand, can he really go on living alone? I just don't know what to say, so I duck out of replying.

> One of my clients has admitted to me that as a young man he committed a series of serious sexual offences against boys. Now he is very ill and in fact is dying. He wants to go to the police to 'confess', then to a priest for absolution. He's constantly asking me what I think he ought to do. I just don't know! I'm struggling against revulsion that he did these things and pity for him now that he's old and harmless. It's making me reluctant to have any contact with him, but he's only told me because we've always got on so well.

> Mavis and her husband are both severely physically disabled. Mavis wants a baby. As one of her home helps she keeps looking to me to discuss whether she should or not. I actually don't think it would be right for them because it would be impossible for them to be proper parents. I find I'm constantly making rather negative and discouraging remarks to her and she looks very hurt,but she's asking my opinion, isn't she, so why shouldn't I tell her?

All three of these clients are asking for advice from their carers, but is it appropriate to give it? The short answer is 'probably not'.

We have all been on the receiving end of the sort of advice that begins 'If I were you . . .' The trouble is that the other person is not you. You can never know exactly what their personal history is in every detail. However open we are with other people, there is always something we hold back, or tell in a way that only represents our own point of view, and that could be the very element that changes the whole picture.

However much you empathize with your client, it would be foolish to imagine that you can tell exactly what it is like to be in their situation. Furthermore, the problem is theirs and not yours. Let us suppose that Mavis decides she cannot have a baby because of disapproval from you. In a few years' time, Mavis may feel bitter and resentful and may blame you because it appears as if it was your decision, not hers.

In this kind of situation, you put yourself in a tricky position if you try to offer advice. Giving advice means telling people what you think they should do, but telling people what to do is not likely to be helpful to them in the long term. A much better tactic is to help them work through the problem so that they come to a decision themselves. The clutch of skills used to do this is usually described as *counselling*.

You should not be put off by the knowledge that people can and do train for many years to become counsellors, or that some of these are professional people with elaborate qualifications. Counselling is certainly a skilled task for which aptitude, training and experience will help, especially when dealing with people whose problems are profound. Most of the issues confronting you as a carer will not be of this kind. However, they are likely to be problems where a *counselling approach* will allow you to help the client in a way that leaves you feeling neither ineffectual (like Mr Wallace's home care assistant) nor over-controlling (like Mavis's).

Some people feel that carers should not become involved in counselling because, they say, it is a difficult skill to acquire and practise. Some clients, they claim, present such intractable problems that only the most experienced and highly trained counsellor can expect to help. It is absolutely true that counselling clients, for instance with serious mental disturbance, or with a long-standing behaviour problem, is indeed a taxing task needing lengthy training. However, simple counselling skills are and should be within the grasp of *most* carers. Whether you like it or not, you will constantly face situations where clients ask you for the kind of help which needs a counselling approach. If you feel you are getting into deep water, then the rule is to ask for help from someone with more experience and training.

What is counselling?

Counselling helps people to help themselves. This may mean:

- supporting them – for instance, through the turmoil and upset of a bereavement or through a difficult period of adjustment to change.
- helping them find a solution to a problem, or to make a decision – for instance, whether to sell their house and move into care.
- helping them understand their own past or present behaviour – for instance, why they always get upset when a particular member of their family visits them, or when they have a conversation with another client or member of staff.

Perhaps you are lucky enough to have had experience yourself of being on the receiving end of helpful counselling from a friend or colleague. If so, it is highly likely that your counsellor had certain characteristics which research has shown are shared by most effective counsellors.

First, such people are not at all interested in *controlling* or dominating other people. Instead, they want to help people use their own resources to find solutions to problems. Good counsellors convey obvious warmth, friendliness and concern, and they also appear strong and self-confident. Strength is an important quality because it suggests that you are in control of your own feelings and can therefore help others. Perhaps an even better phrase would be 'quiet strength' which involves the kind of inner strength that does not overwhelm others. Good counsellors are genuinely interested in other people, are skilled at conveying this and can prompt people to talk by using the kind of body language and questioning described earlier in this chapter.

An effective counsellor also stops herself from judging other people. Here is an experienced professional counsellor describing how this works in practice and why it is so important:

> In my personal life I have all kinds of opinions and prejudices just like everyone else, but I leave them behind when I am working with clients. It is true that I specialize in working with people who have got themselves into dreadful messes one way or another; perhaps they have abused their children, got into appalling debt, become homeless, and so on. People sometimes ask me how I can do this work without thinking or saying 'what an idiot'. But the fact is, the snap judgement is easy; anyone can make it. The real question is always 'why did this happen?', or 'what was it in your life that created this situation?', or 'what's stopping you changing?'. Most of my clients know perfectly

well how society at large regards them, and their self-esteem is already at rock bottom. For me to help them, they must trust me. They will only trust me if I am completely and utterly unshockable, tolerant and non-judgemental. While I'm working with a client my aims are, first, to understand the world as they see it, and second, to help them find positive alternatives that will work for them.

It is unlikely that in your work as a carer you will need to help people with such serious difficulties. However, the need to stay 'non-judgemental' is just as important in counselling people facing any problem which they bring to you for help. Perhaps you have some experience yourself of being on the receiving end of clumsy attempts at counselling, when the other person has tired quickly of listening to you and told you to 'pull yourself together' or to 'snap out of it'. If so, you will know how small it makes you feel and how immediately it destroys the possibility of exploring your feelings further with that person or of looking to them for further help.

Another feature of counselling is that it can only happen if the client wants it. There is no way that you can oblige a client to accept counselling if he or she opposes the idea. This may seem an obvious enough principle, but it is one you may find it surprisingly difficult to accept in practice. The reason is that you may have been drawn to the job of caring by your wish to be helpful to other people. When you see a client faced by a serious dilemma, or overwhelmed by the events in her life, it can be hard to have your offers of counselling help refused, as this carer describes here:

> I was taken on as an escort for a charity that provided holidays for disabled people. My client was a nice young woman with multiple sclerosis in an advanced stage. She had effectively been abandoned by her husband, but couldn't take this in. She kept asking me to ring him for her. At first I did, but he was very abusive and it was clear that he didn't want to talk to me or to her because he regarded the marriage as having ended. We spent a whole ten days together and I kept making opportunities for her to talk to me about her marriage, but she just wasn't having it. In the end she was very snappy and told me to mind my own business. I was very sorry as it was so clear to me that she urgently needed help in coming to terms with what had happened as well as making decisions about her life.

A more subtle form of the same problem may be that by your own skill in getting people to talk, you may produce a rush of confidences that your client later regrets making. This is why you must be very clear at the beginning that the client really welcomes the whole process and is taking part entirely at her own choice.

It will help both your client and you if you also hold clearly in your own mind and explain to your client that the counselling process (and indeed everything else in your dealings with the client) is completely confidential. You should never tell anyone else about counselling conversations with clients without their express permission. The reason is that clients must feel absolute trust that what they tell you will go no further. Without this trust it will be difficult for them to be candid, and candour is usually essential in getting to grips with the problem. It may happen that you feel you need to consult someone more senior about a client. In this case you can either do so without revealing identifying details, or you can ask the client's permission first. Your own employer may have rules on this issue. If so, you should make sure that you and your client know what they are. Whatever your employer's rules, the basic principle is the same. If there are colleagues who need to share the client's secrets, then the client should be aware of these rules before you start the process. In that way he or she will be able to make a better decision about whether to take part or not. (See also page 42 for more on confidentiality.)

Counselling is about identifying the underlying problem rather than just looking at the surface symptoms. For instance, perhaps Mrs A has allowed her room to become spectacularly untidy when it is normally neat. Maybe there is a simple explanation: she has been ill and unable to do even the most basic cleaning for herself. If there is no obvious explanation, it may be worth asking some questions to see if you can find out what the true problem is. Possibly she is depressed and lonely and her untidy room is a symbol of the mess she feels her life is in. Mr B refuses his food and denies that he is hungry. He is steadily losing weight, but there is no obvious physical cause for his loss of appetite. It may help to find out if he is troubled by problems which could be helped by a counselling approach, as in this case:

> Mrs —— had been one of my clients for some years and I went to her home four times a week. Gradually I began to notice

that she looked uneasy and not very welcoming. At first I
thought I'd done something to offend her, but then sensed that
there might be another cause. One day I made her a cup of tea
and one for myself and said 'I've been meaning to have a
chat – you don't seem quite yourself. Is it something I've done?'
At first she didn't respond, but when I persisted gently, she
suddenly burst into tears and told me that she'd developed
urinary incontinence, and dreaded that I could smell it because
she had such difficulties trying to wash her clothing. She had
been too ashamed to tell me. It was a wonderful example of
how useful counselling can be. We had a long talk, she agreed
to see her GP and the problem was actually under control
within a few weeks.

The counselling process

Full-scale counselling normally goes through a number of phases:

Getting to know the client

You are building the relationship at this point, asking questions, and,
if it seems appropriate, perhaps telling the client something about
your own background, establishing trust and friendliness. At this
stage you can say things like: 'Shall we have a chat? You don't seem
too happy', or 'Would you like to talk about the problem of X and
Y'. If the client says 'no', then of course you have to stop at this stage.

Exploring the problem

Here you are asking more questions, collecting more information
and trying to look at the problem from every angle. You might try
questions such as 'When did this first start to bother you?' or 'What
is it about the problem that worries you most?', reflecting and
summarizing as described in the section on empathy (page 75).

It is often particularly useful to explore the pros and cons of, say,
a particular decision at this stage. What would be the advantages
and disadvantages of following a particular course of action? What
does the client feel matters most to her? For instance, if Mr Wallace

(page 83) is still uncertain about whether to carry on living alone or to move into care, you could discuss with him which he feels is more important, his physical safety or living in his own home. To do this you would need to ask him how many times he has had falls and how serious he thinks they are, as well as asking him how well he feels he copes with the other aspects of looking after himself.

It may be that he does not fall often and that arranging for him to have sticks or a walking frame might be a better solution than the drastic step of selling his home. On the other hand, if worry about his health has become a serious concern then the sacrifice of his independence might be better than carrying on alone. But all kinds of other solutions might emerge at this point – for example, an alarm system; a joint household with a friend or family member; or grab rails in strategic places. But in the end, the solution has to be one that he feels comfortable with and that he has found for himself. You may do this so skilfully that the client may be quite unaware that you have had anything to do with the decision at all, as in this case:

> I was assigned to a young family on a short-term basis where the wife was being treated in hospital for cancer. The husband didn't know whether to tell his wife and their children the diagnosis or not. We had several long conversations where we went through all the arguments. I just gently kept asking him questions, rephrasing, summarizing, and so on, as I'd been taught on our training course. At the end of it, he suddenly said: 'Yes, I see now I must tell her. I've suddenly got decisive – I don't know what was wrong with me before!' I don't think he realized that I'd had the slightest hand in it, but I didn't mind. He'd made what he felt was the right decision and that was the important thing.

Challenging and influencing

Most of the counselling you are likely to be involved with as a carer will probably stop at the second stage of exploring the problem. However, with more experience and training, you may be able to embark on the third stage, where you try to get the client to look again at problems which seem to be stuck in a groove. Here you are suggesting that there might be other points of view, and other solutions. Here is one carer, now running her own care home after many years as a care assistant, describing one case in which she used this technique successfully:

> I have many clients who seem to go round and round on one particular issue. The local authority in my previous job sent me on a training course which included counselling and this gave me a lot of confidence to try these approaches. I remember one elderly woman client who was very bitter about the fact that her family hardly ever came to see her. Her anger was really burning her up. I made time to see her every day to talk about it over a period of ten days. We covered a lot of ground and eventually I started saying little things like 'Imagine you were your son, what would you be saying about coming here?', and 'How do you think your behaviour when he *does* visit affects him?', and 'What do you think would persuade him to visit you more?'. In this way I gradually got her to see that one reason they didn't visit was that she spent the whole visit trying to make them feel guilty about their failure to offer her a home with them. The visits were so unpleasant for them that they had simply stopped coming. In the end, she did see the problem differently and wrote [her son] a jolly good letter. This brought him in and she did manage to put the whole thing on a completely different footing.

Making the changes

In the final stage of counselling, the client has decided to change, or has made a decision, but will now need supporting. Here, your comments and questions will be along these lines: 'How do you feel it is going?', 'What problems are emerging and what should we do about them?'. Your efforts here will include the need to withdraw from the counselling role, even though your professional relationship may continue as before.

Summary

This chapter has been about the importance of good communication skills: listening, talking and body language. Proper communication alerts you early to problems with clients. It means you can represent their interests better, and gives you the satisfaction of knowing that you are helping meet their needs. Good communication is never easy because lack of time, lack of privacy, differences in culture and problems of physical or mental disability can all get in the way. Successful communication involves developing the skills of empathy, essential if you are going to help by giving clients advice or by guiding them, by means of the counselling approach, towards finding the best solutions to their problems themselves.

6

Dealing with emergencies

All carers have to be capable of dealing competently with emergencies. Whether you work in people's own homes, or in institutions, you may have to give first aid, deal with a fire, cope with the aftermath of a burglary or call the emergency services. In any of these situations you will need to know how to look after yourself and how to do your best for other people. There is no substitute for practical training in these matters, but the aim of this chapter is to introduce you to some of the main emergencies that it is possible you might meet in your work, how to prevent them happening at all, and the main principles of dealing with them if they do.

Being safety-conscious

All employers and employees have responsibility under the Health and Safety at Work Act to prevent risks to everyone's health and safety by, for instance, keeping to safety rules, wearing protective clothing where it is prudent, not tampering with equipment, and reporting anything that seems unsafe. Employers are expected to appoint a 'health and safety' representative, as well as trained first-aiders, and should provide everyone with health and safety information and training – for example, fire drills.

Most employers take this duty seriously, not least because they fear the prosecution and insurance claims that would result from neglect. Even so, in day-to-day terms, it is you, not your employer, whose responsibility it is to interpret the detail of the health and safety policy so that both you and your clients are protected from risk as far as possible.

The best protection of all is to train yourself to be safety-conscious at all times. Is that carpet wearing out so that frayed threads might trip someone? If so, report it straight away. How do you feel about fire drills? The only sensible way to regard them is as a serious rehearsal for what you would need to do in a real fire. Do you know how to report an accident? If not, find out. Are those chemicals used for cleaning stored where they cannot be easily spilled or mistaken for harmless fluids? If not, put them in a safer place. Keeping a constant eye open for hazards is one of the best preventive measures of all. Thinking that they are someone else's responsibility is one of the ways in which preventable accidents happen.

Make sure that you always carry or have available a handy list of emergency numbers. This should include some or all of the following:

- client's doctor
- council/client's/organization's/emergency plumbing, electrical and security services
- local police
- Electricity Board
- Gas Board
- Water Board
- client's next of kin
- your manager's work and home numbers.

Calling the emergency services

The emergency services – fire, ambulance and police – are there to provide prompt and skilled help for the kind of situation where there is no DIY solution. You should not feel any hesitation about calling them; they are trained to judge the seriousness of the problem. So never feel that you might be wasting their time – leave them to decide how to react.

Your employer may have a particular policy about making 999 calls. For instance, in a residential home or hospital, you may have to route them through the switchboard or dial a special number on your own internal system. However, most employers will encourage you to use your initiative and discretion and the basic rule here is: *when in doubt, ring 999.*

The main situations in which you will need to make an emergency call are:

Medical: difficulty in breathing
                    severe bleeding
                    unconsciousness
                    suspected heart attack
                    serious burns
Fire: any fire that has taken hold, including
                    chimney fires, frying pan fires that have taken
                    hold in kitchens; smoke or fire alarm being set
                    off.
Other problems: Gas leaks, water bursts, intruders, burglars or
                    suspicion of any other serious crime.

Emergency calls are free; you don't need money to dial 999 from a public phone. What happens is as follows. You dial 999 and the operator says 'Emergency, which service do you require?' You reply 'ambulance' or 'fire' or 'police'. The operator will pass messages to the other services if all three are needed. She then asks you what number you are calling from; this is in case you are cut off. You are then connected to the emergency service controller who again will ask the number of your phone. Be prepared now to describe, accurately and concisely

- what the incident is
- where it has happened and how the emergency services can find their way
- how many people are involved, their age, sex and condition, any special problems – for instance, whether breathing apparatus will be needed if there are fumes.

Do not put the phone down until the operator does.

While you are waiting for the emergency services to arrive, do anything you can to help them gain access quickly – for instance, putting on all the front lights if it is dark, opening doors, sending someone to look out for them and guide them.

Fire

It is sad to say that fire is a real danger for most carers' clients. The worse off your clients are, the more likely they are to have makeshift electrical wiring and to keep their homes warm with the least safe forms of heating such as open fires and paraffin heaters. When clients are physically disabled it will be harder for them to escape from a burning building safely. Elderly people sometimes lose their sense of smell so do not get early warning of a fire. When they are confused or mentally handicapped, it is more likely that they will forget the cigarette smouldering next to an armchair which starts a fire many hours later when the client is asleep. Physically disabled people can have problems which mean that they may unintentionally drop a lighted match or have difficulty bending to clear away the apparently harmless rubbish which can become the centre of a blaze if a fire breaks out.

Precautions against fire

Fortunately, there are plenty of sensible precautions which you can take with your clients or on their behalf.

Open fires should always have spark or fire guards to prevent sparks jumping out and smouldering on rugs and carpets. Some clients like fire guards but then use them to dry or air clothing and tea towels. Try to discourage this by pointing out that scorched clothing can sometimes go from scorching to flames in a few seconds.

Women clients often wear loose nightdresses, but these can be dangerous if the client also has an open fire or paraffin heater because the clothing can flap dangerously close to the flames. Adult nightwear is not generally made from fire-retardant fabric, but persuading clients to wear pyjamas instead will help to cut down the risks. Natural fibres are generally less flammable than synthetic ones.

Paraffin and portable gas heaters are best treated as if they were fixed permanently, and should be placed where they are least likely to get knocked over. A paraffin heater, particularly, should *never* be moved when it is alight.

Cigarettes and matches are one of the main causes of fires. The reason is that cigarettes and matches are often not completely extinguished; the smouldering butts may be tossed into a plastic bin containing waste paper, may be ground into a carpet or thrown out of a window. If the butt or match is still alight, it may cause serious problems. It is unlikely that you will be able to persuade people to give up smoking, but the main reason why smokers dispose of their butts and matches carelessly is that there is no proper ashtray within easy reach, so the solution to this fire risk is to make sure that there are plenty of heavy, large, generously rimmed ashtrays everywhere. They should be emptied frequently into a fireproof container and smokers and their visitors encouraged to use them.

Smoking in bed should always be discouraged. A smoker who has fallen asleep with a lit cigarette in his or her hand may easily set fire to bedclothes with tragic results. Warning clients of the risk needs to be done with some skill, as this home care assistant comments:

> I'm a smoker myself, so perhaps that makes it a bit easier, but I really do a big number on the danger of having a last fag in bed. As I say to them, it could literally be your last fag! There's no point in trying to make rules as such because all you get, even in eighty-year-olds, is a teenager-like determination to outwit you and be a daredevil. So the way I approach it is to say that if you fancy a cigarette before going to bed, have it downstairs, stub it out in a nice big ashtray and then go to bed with a clear conscience and clean teeth! That *seems* to work.

The kitchen is another prime source of fire danger. Cookers should be treated with respect and pan handles always turned inwards. Encourage clients to develop a routine to check that the main switch on an electric cooker is in the 'off' position when not in use and that all the gas taps are properly turned off on a gas cooker.

Boiling fat is a frequent source of kitchen fires. The rules here are never to fill a pan more than one-third full and never to leave a chip pan unattended. Watch the fat for any signs of the blue or black smoke which indicates that the danger point has been reached when, if the heat under the pan is not reduced, the fat could burst into flames. A fire blanket stored in an accessible place is an excellent safety precaution in a kitchen. If a fire should break out, the blanket can be used to smother the flames safely. Fire blankets are not expensive. Some councils will purchase them for disabled clients living in their own homes as a way of reducing the risk of fire, and of helping preserve the independence of clients who wish to continue cooking for themselves.

Faulty plugs, sockets, appliances and wiring can also cause fires. You are unlikely to be able to foresee problems in a faulty appliance, but the danger from wires and overloaded sockets is usually all too visible:

> One of my clients lives in a 1920s semi which was originally

owned by her parents. It's had nothing spent on it since. When I first went there I discovered that there were hardly any electrical sockets, and the ones she did have were unbelievably dangerous. In her lounge she had a single round-pin socket with three adaptors permanently in place running her TV, electric fire, a table lamp and a radio! The cables were trailing everywhere and very worn, you could see the bare wire on several of them.

This situation was a classic recipe for fire. Sockets should have at most one adaptor, cables should be tucked around walls, faulty flex replaced and a wiring system untouched since the 1920s should certainly be checked by a qualified electrician. You should also do what you can to persuade clients to get into a routine of unplugging television sets when they are not in use, as colour sets in particular can cause a fire even when the set is switched off but still plugged into the socket.

Several recent public tragedies have made us all aware of the danger that can lurk in piles of rubbish. Left to dry out, especially if they include a combination of paper and grease, as much household rubbish does, they can become dangerous fire hazards. In institutions this is easily tackled; there are usually plenty of large covered bins and the only problem is to motivate people to use them. In clients' own homes great tact may be needed:

Several of my clients are terrible hoarders. I have one who keeps and washes old tins, and three or four who 'save' newspapers. One explained to me that as a girl, newsprint was valuable; you tore it up into little squares for the lavatory, you used it to line boots in the winter, to clean windows and in dozens of other ways to save money, and now she can't get out of the habit. The scouts used to collect bundles of it from her, but they've given that up, so now she has wobbling bundles of newspaper everywhere. I explained to her that I thought some old newspaper could be jolly useful, but she didn't need it all and it was a fire risk because, first, it would burn too easily, and second, she had so many piles of it in her hall on the stairs and in the kitchen it would prevent her getting out quickly. I let her mull it over for a few weeks and then I casually suggested that she kept a few bundles, but that I could organize the council to do a special collection for recycling. I knew that would appeal to her thrifty nature and it did. She agreed straight away.

When a fire does break out, the main danger to people is usually from smoke and fumes. Few victims actually burn to death but many suffocate. The reason is that so much cheap modern furniture is filled with foam which gives off dangerous fumes when it burns. If these fumes fill a room, anyone inside will die within minutes. This type of foam is now illegal in new furniture, but much of the old type is still around. It makes sense to keep all furniture well away from direct heat, including cigarettes.

Apart from doing what you can to minimize the risk of fire from cigarettes, matches, cookers, electrical equipment, rubbish and foam-filled furniture, you can also make sure you are familiar with any simple fire-fighting equipment that is available. Residential homes and hospitals will have fire extinguishers of various kinds, including the fire blankets already mentioned. There are strict regulations about fire doors. These are heavy, self-closing doors which can help prevent the spread of fire from one part of a large building to another. They should always remain closed, even if you are tempted to prop them open for wheelchair or trolley access.

When you work in clients' own homes you can copy the useful precaution of fire doors by encouraging clients to close all doors between rooms at night. In the event of a fire this would have the same desirable effect of containing the fire, especially the smoke and fumes. Fire and smoke alarms and sprinklers are also a necessity in residential homes and hospitals; make sure you know how to activate the fire alarm if you work in an institutional setting, and try to persuade clients to invest in a smoke alarm if you work in their own homes. Simple smoke alarms are cheap to buy and easy to install and run.

When you have fire drills, use the opportunity to practise the techniques that you would need in an actual fire. Some employers go to a lot of trouble to simulate the real situation, turning off the lights and using 'safe' smoke to bring home the need, for instance, to memorize the layout of rooms and the location of fire exits so that you can escape by feeling your way along the walls. This is a useful rehearsal, even though you sincerely hope, as everyone does, that you will never have to use this knowledge and skill for real. Fire drills always include gathering at agreed 'assembly points'. This is to make sure that everyone is accounted for. In an actual fire, this helps identify missing people quickly and to pinpoint the part of the building they are likely to be in.

Remember, too, that in a real fire at night, there will be no lights. It will be frighteningly dark and smoky. Memorizing the escape route is doubly important, and so is making sure that nothing ever blocks the main exits. In their own homes, discourage clients from leaving shopping trolleys, wheelchairs or other bulky objects where they might block hall, stairs and landing and introduce them to the idea that the quickest way to get out of a fire is to work your way along the walls of a room.

Dealing with a fire

If the worst happens and a fire does break out, you need to know what to do. Clear, swift thinking is essential.

A chip-pan fire can be put out in its earliest stages by throwing a fire blanket or damp tea-towel over it in order to smother the flames. Never try to move the pan. The movement will fan the flames, putting you at grave risk of burning your face and hair and splashing boiling fat all over your body.

If a fire has taken hold in a room, the most important thing to do is to guarantee your own safety first, then to warn other people in the building and phone the emergency services. Acts of attempted heroism – for instance, dashing into the burning building to rescue others – may be well intentioned but they are utterly foolish. You need special training, protective clothing and breathing apparatus to attempt such a rescue; this is exactly why fire brigades are the only people who should do it.

If you work in a residential home or hospital, your fire drill will include techniques for getting disabled and bedridden people out of the building quickly. It is important to practise these techniques; they have enabled many carers to save innumerable lives by swift emergency evacuation before the fire has spread. Even the simple act of closing all doors behind you as you leave could help save a life. Never use the lifts in this situation; electrical equipment is usually the first to be put out of action. Using a lift could mean being cut off from help.

The most dangerous situation of all where fire is concerned is to be trapped inside the building with escape routes cut off by fire or fumes. In this case, you and any clients involved should put sheets, blankets or coats against the top and bottom of the closed door to keep out smoke, and call for help from the window.

Gas

> One of my clients has rapidly developing senile dementia. I came into her house one day and found it smelling strongly of gas. She was wandering in the garden quite unaware that she'd put the gas cooker on without lighting it. It was the most frightening situation I've ever had to face, but fortunately I only really felt frightened afterwards; at the time I was totally calm!

What would you have done if you had been in this situation? The procedure is similar to that for fire – the first rule is to protect yourself, so if there is any real danger of explosion, leave the building immediately and raise the alarm. Where the danger is not so acute, this is what to do:

- Turn off the gas; if there is a leak rather than simply an open tap on a cooker, turn off the main gas supply to the house. This is normally a large lever situated in the meter cupboard and marked with 'on' and 'off' positions.
- Open the windows and doors.
- Do not use any electrical switches, as even tiny sparks could make the gas explode.
- Stop anyone in the area smoking.
- Give first aid to anyone who is unconscious from fumes.
- Call for help. In the case of a gas leak, ring the Gas Board, who will have an emergency number prominently displayed in your local phone book.

Medical emergencies

You may well be confronted by an emergency where the client's life is threatened. You are likely to feel frightened at the time and to worry afterwards about whether you did the right thing. These are perfectly normal reactions:

> The meals on wheel people had just brought Mr —— 's dinner

and he was eating it quite happily when suddenly he choked on a piece of meat. It was no good running to anyone else for help, he was turning blue and there was only me there to help. I bent him over and thumped his back but it was no good, I could hear his attempts at gasping getting fainter and fainter. On television I'd seen the 'bear hug' [abdominal thrust technique, see page 107 demonstrated, so I got behind him and did what I remembered. The meat came shooting out. In a few seconds he was fine, but what if he'd died? What if I'd broken his ribs? He is a thin, frail old man and I sometimes dream that the whole thing is happening again except that I can't get the meat out. It was horrible. At the same time I know I saved his life and his family have made a great fuss of me, but I feel uncomfortable about that, too!

A client had a heart attack while I was with her. I called the ambulance and I managed to comfort her, but all the time I was terrified that she'd die and somehow it would be my fault. I know now that I did the right thing, but it took me a while to settle down afterwards.

Employers normally have their own policies about first aid. For instance, some employers insist that if a client falls you do nothing other than call for help; this is based on the common but false idea that it is better to do nothing than to risk making a difficult situation worse. Actually the reverse is true – in most of the common life-threatening emergencies, it is almost always better to do something than nothing. Only you can decide how to react if your work presents you with the dilemma of whether to help a client in contradiction of your employer's guidelines.

Many employers take the more sensible and helpful attitude that first-aid training is the best way to make sure that their staff know how to react. Even if your employer does not provide first-aid training, it is worth seeing if you can arrange it for yourself. The main skills can be acquired in a single two- to three-hour session and are not difficult to learn. Many organizations, including the Red Cross, St John, St Andrew and local hospitals now run such sessions where, for a nominal fee, you can learn what to do in an emergency.

The most important techniques are the ones called *cardio-pulmonary resuscitation* (CPR). You will probably know them as 'the kiss of life' and 'heart massage'. Both these popular terms are misleading: there is no 'kiss' involved in mouth-to-mouth breathing and 'massage' creates completely the wrong impression of the hard work involved in giving chest compressions. It is better to refer to them by their correct name, CPR. The best way to learn CPR is to go to a class where you can see it skilfully demonstrated and practise it on a manikin, a life-sized dummy specially designed for this training. Normally at these classes you can also learn the techniques for dealing with choking and for placing a casualty in the 'recovery position'.

There is no attempt in this chapter to give you detailed instructions in the major first-aid techniques. For that you will need to attend a class. However, the following sections will give you some basic guidelines on what to do in some of the most common medical emergencies.

The same fundamental rule applies here as to any emergency: do not put yourself at risk. If you become the cause of another accident you cannot help the injured or ill client and also create more problems for other rescuers.

Assess the situation quickly but calmly. What can you observe that will help you find out what has happened? For instance, if you discover an unconscious client lying in bed, are there open pill bottles which suggest an overdose? Is there a smell of vomit which might imply that the client has choked? If a client has fallen, what can you see around her which could explain the reason? Is the floor slippery? Has she been trying to change a lightbulb by standing on a rickety chair?

Now you can decide how to give help. Usually in a serious emergency it is better to give first aid *before* calling for help. The reason is that there is often very little time left in which to save the client's life. For example, let us suppose that you discover that a client has stopped breathing. There are now only three to four minutes before irreversible brain damage sets in. If you go off to fetch help, the client could be dead by the time you return. So give first aid, and go for help only *when it is safe to leave the client*.

Unconsciousness

A client may become unconscious for a whole range of reasons – heart attack, stroke, choking, poisoning, head injury, electric shock, bleeding, fainting and epilepsy. Unconsciousness is always a major emergency. The reason is that when we are unconscious, all our muscles relax. Particularly important here is the tongue, which falls to the back of the throat and, if the casualty is on his or her back, will block the airway. You may sometimes hear this described as 'swallowing the tongue'. Unless the airway is opened, the casualty will die from suffocation within a few minutes. People who are otherwise fit and healthy frequently die for this reason, so it is important to know how to open the airway.

- First, check that the casualty really is unconscious by shaking her shoulder gently and shouting 'Are you all right?'. A person who is not deeply unconscious will respond. If there is no response, assume that the casualty is unconscious.
- Now you must open the airway. You do this by lifting the chin forwards with one hand while pressing the forehead back with the other hand. This lifts the tongue off the back of the throat (see Figure 3).
- Check the casualty's breathing by looking for chest movements, listening for breath sounds and feeling breath on your own cheek.

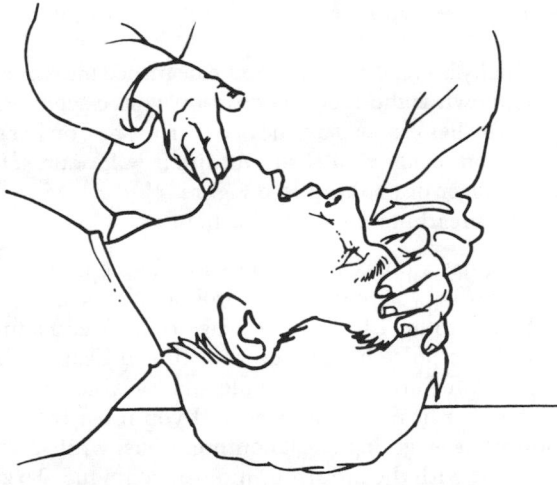

Figure 3 How to open the airway

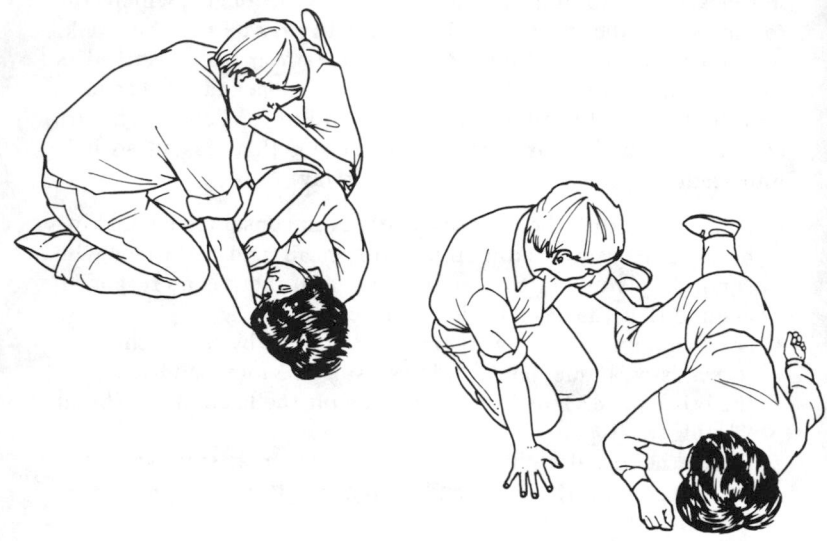

Figure 4 The recovery position

- If the casualty is breathing, she should be turned into the safe stable position known as the 'recovery position' where her airway is kept open and she lies propped by one of her arms, half on her stomach. This position means that if she vomits it will drain safely away with no danger of choking (see Figure 4).
- Check her breathing again, go for help.

If breathing has stopped then you should give mouth-to-mouth breathing by sealing your own mouth around the casualty's and using your out-breath to breath into her lungs twice (see Figure 5).

Now check her pulse by putting your fingers against the groove in her neck between the Adam's apple and the voicebox. If there is no pulse then her heart has stopped and you must try to keep her circulation going by giving chest compressions, while also keeping breathing going with the mouth-to-mouth technique. To give chest compressions, you must:

- keep her airway open.

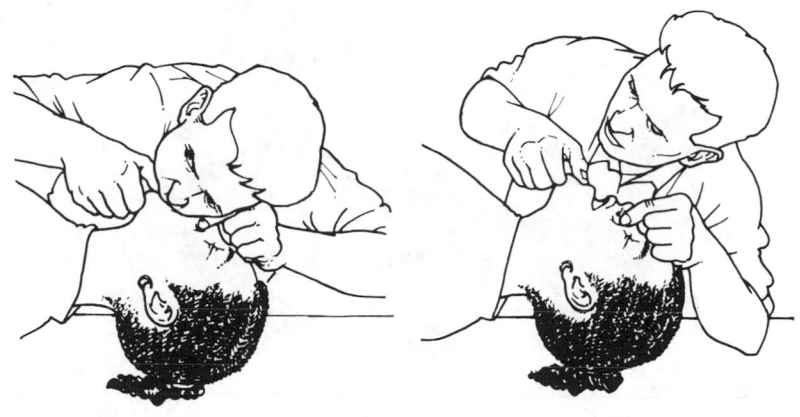

Figure 5 Mouth-to-mouth breathing

- rhythmically press down hard but not jerkily on her breastbone, keeping your own elbows straight and hands clasped, at the rate of about eight a minute.
- combine this with mouth-to-mouth resuscitation. The usual pattern is to give two breaths followed by fifteen compressions and to keep going either until breathing and pulse restart or until skilled medical help arrives.

When you have never had any practical training in CPR this sounds complicated, but with training and practice it can become second nature. Here is how one care assistant found she could call on her first-aid training:

I was serving tea in the dining room when one of the ladies just keeled right over with no apparent warning. There was pandemonium and the other residents were crying and frightened. I felt utterly calm because I knew my CPR routine backwards as I'd only just done the training. I got her on the

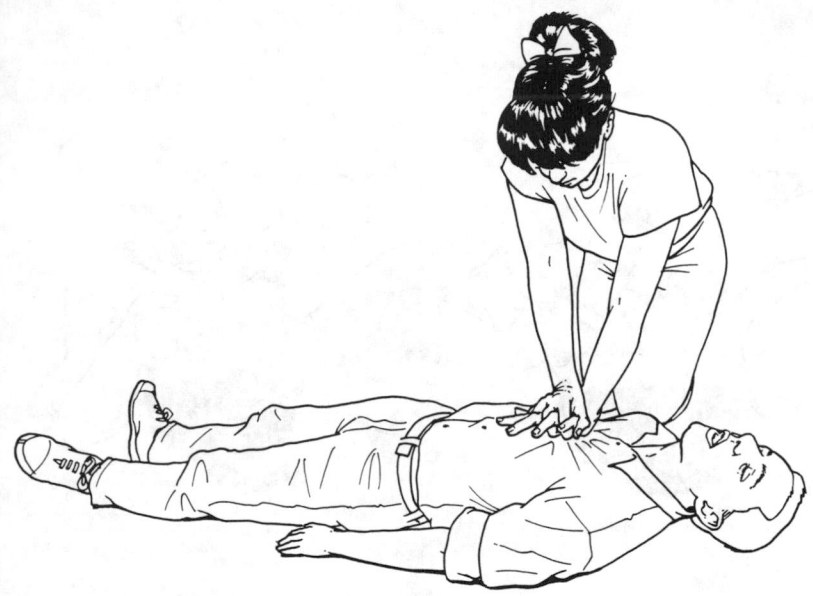

Figure 6 Chest compressions

floor, told Joan [another care assistant] to call an ambulance
and get the residents out of the way, opened her airway, checked
her breathing, did the two breaths, checked pulse, no pulse
and started CPR. I worked on her for ten minutes – it was
incredibly tiring – until the ambulance came and they took
over. They had a defibrillator [a piece of equipment which gives
an electric jolt to the heart] and revived her in the ambulance.
She eventually returned to the home and lived a really full life
for a good year afterwards when she had another attack and
died in her sleep. I'm sure she would have died the first time
if I hadn't known what to do: I feel really proud of myself.

Choking

A choking client is at risk of death unless someone can help her
dislodge the obstruction in her airway. She will be frightened and
may be turning blue. This is what to do:

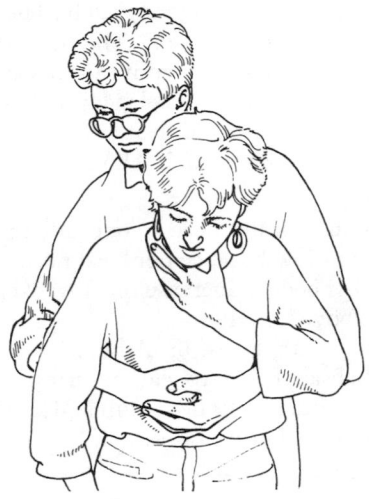

Figure 7 The abdominal thrust

- Reassure her, get her to bend over, as gravity helps.
- Encourage her to cough.
- Give several sharp blows between her shoulder blades.
- If this fails, the abdominal thrust technique may work. Stand behind the client, putting both of your arms around her, with your hands clasped into a fist, now pull sharply inwards and upwards. This forces air out of the gullet and often dislodges the obstruction (see Figure 7). This technique is best learnt at a class before trying to apply it.

Bleeding

Heavy bleeding can lead to shock and may be fatal unless it is stopped. Use a clean pad (a handkerchief, tea towel or sheet will do) and press hard against the wound. If possible, lift the injured part higher than the level of the chest to slow down the flow of blood.

Shock

The word 'shock' has a different medical meaning from its everyday use, where it simply means a fright. Shock is a serious condition where the body reacts to an emergency such as heart attack, a fall, a serious burn or an allergic reaction. The result is that the brain and other vital organs are suddenly deprived of blood, and the casualty will be pale, cold, clammy and will feel giddy and sick. Serious shock may lead to unconsciousness and death.

This is what to do if a client is in shock:

- Reassure her.
- Lay her down and turn her head to one side in case she is sick, but do not use a pillow because her head needs to be kept lower than the rest of her body to increase the flow of blood to her brain.
- Raise her legs above her chest.
- Cover her lightly with a coat or blanket.
- Do not give her anything to eat or drink – if she becomes unconscious this could make her vomit and may also prevent her being given an anaesthetic in hospital.

Heart attack

In Britain we are in the unenviable position of still being near the top of the world league for heart disease. It is an epidemic so common that we forget that heart disease was unknown a hundred years ago and that most doctors had never seen a case involving it. It is now clear that the causes of heart disease are smoking, our diet of fatty, highly-refined foods, alcohol and lack of exercise. Heredity is also a factor for some people.

All these elements are so common that it is very likely that your clients will include people with heart disease and you may well have to cope with clients who develop the symptoms of a heart attack while you are with them.

This is what to do if a client seems to be having a heart attack:

- Recognize the symptoms for what they are. They include
  - Crushing, vice-like pain in the chest which may spread to jaw, shoulders and arms and hardly ever starts suddenly; it usually develops over several minutes or even hours.
  - Feeling sick.
  - Feeling giddy and breathless.
  - Clammy skin.
- Dial 999 and ask for an ambulance saying that you suspect a heart attack.

- Reassure the client saying that help is coming.
- Keep the client comfortable in a half-sitting, half-lying position and do not give anything to eat or drink.
- If he becomes unconscious or stops breathing you will have to give CPR.

Heart attack victims are at greatest risk of death within the first hour of their symptoms developing. So the sooner you get a client to hospital, where special equipment and drugs are available, the better his chances of recovery.

Burns and scalds

Serious burns are life-threatening because so much fluid can leak from them that shock develops, or infection can set in which overwhelms the body's defences. A burn is serious when it is bigger than one square inch, does not hurt because it is so deep that it has destroyed nerve endings and when the skin looks waxy and charred. Burns and scalds are also serious when they are associated with shock, unconsciousness or where throat and mouth are affected and swelling may affect breathing.

This is what to do:

- *Where clothing is on fire*
  - Put the flames out by throwing a bucket of water over the casualty or wrapping her in a coat and laying her down quickly to prevent the torch-like effect that flames can have on a standing casualty.
  - Do not try to remove burnt clothing as you may remove skin with it.
- *Cool the burnt or scalded area continuously in cold water* to reduce the heat of the skin.
- *Cover the burn* with a clean, non-fluffy fabric and tie or pin it in place. Cling film has been used successfully to improvise a dressing in some kitchen accidents.
- *Call an ambulance.*
- *Treat for shock* and reassure the client.
- *Be prepared* to give CPR if the casualty becomes unconscious.

Electric shock

A frayed flex, a faulty fitting on a lightbulb, a damaged switch can all lead to serious accidents because the electric current can cause deep burns as it passes through the body and may even affect the heart or the part of the brain that controls breathing.

Here is what to do if a client has an electric shock:

- Do not touch her until you have separated her safely from the current. Do this by switching off the power at the socket or main fuse box.
- If this is impossible, stand on something that will insulate you – a rubber mat, pile of dry newspapers or dry clothing – and use a stick, stool, umbrella or looped sheet to pull her away from the source of the current.
- If she is unconscious open her airway and check for breathing (see page 104) and give CPR if necessary.
- Cover the burn with a dressing.
- Treat her for shock.
- Call an ambulance: it is vital that anyone who has had a serious electric shock should have a medical check as their injuries may be more severe than they seem.

Poisoning

Poisoning may result from a client's attempt at suicide or from an accidental overdose, from drinking too much or from unintended contact with one of the many dangerous chemicals most kitchens and gardens now contain.

Here is what to do:

- Do not put yourself at risk – for instance, by contaminating yourself with chemicals or entering a garage filled with carbon monoxide.
- Look for the evidence that will tell you what has happened: empty bottles, spilled fluids, a smell of alcohol.
- Put an unconscious casualty in the recovery position and keep checking pulse and breathing. Do not give mouth-to-mouth resuscitation to a casualty who appears to have chemical burns around the mouth, as you could be affected, too.
- Ring for an ambulance, describing what you have seen. If the client has vomited it might be useful to give the crew a sample to take away for analysis.

- Do not encourage a conscious client to be sick as this may make the damage worse by bringing her mouth and throat into contact with the poison again.

Stroke

The symptoms of a stroke may include problems in moving limbs and face on one side of the body, difficulty speaking and breathing as well as unconsciousness.

Here is what to do:

- If the client is unconscious keep her airway open. Turn her into the recovery position and keep checking her breathing and pulse, giving CPR if necessary.
- Send for an ambulance.
- A conscious client should be reassured that help is on its way and should be treated for shock.

Epileptic fits

Epilepsy is caused by an electrical disturbance to the brain. Although frightening for the client, it is not so dangerous as it looks as long as the unconsciousness does not last too long and the client is not injured while falling.

The symptoms include crying out just before the fit begins, unconsciousness followed by stiffening and jerking and noisy or difficult breathing. The body then relaxes and some sufferers may wet or soil themselves as their muscle control goes. Unconsciousness may last a few more minutes.

Epilepsy used to be regarded as a shameful secret because it was quite wrongly linked with mental illness. Today it is responsive to drugs and sufferers are usually more open about it. If you have a client who has epilepsy, you will probably know about it in advance and you may be able to discuss the frequency of any attacks he experiences and how he likes to be treated.

Here is what to do if a client has an epileptic fit:

- Break his fall if you can and move away any heavy furniture that could get in the way during the convulsive stage, but otherwise leave him alone.

- Do not try to put anything in his mouth – this is not necessary and could be dangerous.
- When the jerking is over, turn him into the recovery position.
- As he comes round he will be drowsy and confused, so reassure him and persuade him to rest for at least ten minutes.
- Cover him lightly with a blanket to preserve his dignity, if he has wet or soiled himself.
- Keep any bystanders away.

You do not need to call an ambulance unless he has hurt himself badly in the fall or the unconsciousness continues for a long time, or one fit is followed immediately by several others.

Hypothermia

Elderly clients are especially prone to this condition, which is caused by a sharp fall in body temperature. People at risk will include immobile and undernourished clients so worried about paying their fuel bills that they insist on living in unheated rooms. Public concern about hypothermia has led to Electricity and Gas Boards offering special concessions to elderly people, to charities offering free 'warning' thermometers and to much more vigilance by care staff.

Even so, hypothermia is a constant risk to low-income clients living in their own homes. The symptoms include uncontrollable shivering, skin that feels very cold to your touch, drowsiness, limpness and very slow pulse and breathing rates. In its early stages, hypothermia can be reversed, but if the body temperature drops below 26°C (75°F) it is usually fatal; unconsciousness is followed by the failure of breathing and pulse and the client dies.

Here is what to do if you suspect hypothermia in a client:

- Call an ambulance.
- Warm a bed with an electric blanket or hot water bottle (you may be able to borrow these from neighbours).
- Put her into bed and place a covered hot water bottle in her left armpit to warm her 'core' circulation, but don't use hot water bottles anywhere else as they will draw blood away from her vital organs.
- Reassure her and keep talking to her.

- If she has become cold gradually, then aim to rewarm her gradually: this may take several hours.
- If she has become hypothermic suddenly, for instance by falling in a snowdrift, then you can rewarm her more quickly in a hot bath.
- Give her a hot drink to sip slowly.
- Put an unconscious hypothermic client into the recovery position and keep checking her breathing and pulse.

Falls

Falls are one of the main dangers to confused or physically disabled people. Bones which have become thin and therefore brittle are more likely to break easily and will also take a long time to heal. A client who has fallen may develop shock or pneumonia and die. For all these reasons it is important to put a lot of effort into cutting down the risks of people having falls. The main steps that can be taken will include:

- improving lighting, especially on steps so that clients see hazards clearly
- avoiding loose rugs which can ruck and trip people up
- repairing frayed and worn carpets
- cleaning polished or tiled floors at times when clients are not using them to cut down the chance of clients falling on the slippery surface
- installing ramps and safety rails
- putting rubber safety mats in baths and showers.

In spite of all your precautions, clients may still have occasional falls. Falls worry employers because they fear prosecution by angry relatives, and also because some falls can result in spinal injury which can be made worse by inexpert handling. It is important to make clear that in most of the falls your clients are likely to have there will be no risk of spinal injury, so to do nothing, as some employers nervously advise, is not in the client's best interest.

Straightforward falls are the ones where an unsteady client topples over perhaps while getting into and out of bed or simply when walking.

Here is what to do if a client falls:

- Ask the client what has happened and whether he has any pain; reassure and comfort him.
- Ask someone to help you lift him up and sit him down in a chair.
- If he is shocked, lie him down and treat for shock (page 107).
- If he is unconscious, open his airway, keep it open (page 104) and call for help.
- If a client falls in the bath, call for help if possible, then let out the water and dry the client while he is still in the bath, keeping him covered with towels and a blanket. Don't attempt to lift him out on your own as this is a skilled job for at least two people.

Spinal injury is always a possibility if the client has fallen from a height. If the client is unconscious you should still make the protection of his airway a priority, supporting it until skilled help arrives. Do not attempt to move the client on your own and summon an ambulance as quickly as possible.

Security

Although hospitals and residential homes may sometimes suffer outbreaks of petty thieving, security is usually more of a problem for home care assistants and their clients. This home care assistant tells a typical story:

> When I visited Mrs M that day, I discovered that her home had been ransacked and half her furniture and china stolen. She'd told me a few days before that she'd been visited by a charming 'antiques dealer' who'd paid a lot of money for an old vase and who'd had a good look around by the sound of it, asking to use the loo and so on. I reckoned he'd come back and waited for her to go out. He had driven up a big van, cool as you like, broken in in broad daylight and taken her stuff. She was absolutely heartbroken, so distressed, I just didn't know how to comfort her. The things that had been taken had been in her family for years and I don't think she had any idea how valuable a lot of it was.

Although this tale is all too common, it is important for both you and your client to keep a sense of proportion. Statistics show that elderly people are not actually attacked or robbed any more than any other group, but the way such crimes are reported when they do occur certainly increases their sense of alarm. You can do a lot to calm their fears by helping them to take sensible precautions.

Preventing crime

Encourage clients to invest in mortise locks on front and back doors. The locks should conform to British Standard 3621. Locks that meet this standard will say that they conform to BS3621 on the packaging. Simple window locks or screws for sash windows can make windows more difficult to force. Many clients may leave their key under the mat so that you or neighbours can get in easily, but tell them that this is the first place a burglar looks, and the second place a burglar looks is to see whether the back door key has been left in the lock on the inside, where breaking a pane of glass makes it easy to remove.

A strong door with a good hinge on the inside deters the sort of burglar who specializes in kicking down or axing a door. A door viewer and chain will emphasize to casual callers that the client is cautious. Local old people's charities may be able to help pay for locks, bolts and doors if clients cannot afford to buy them themselves. Outside lights front and back burn very little electricity and will also help deter intruders who rely on darkness to conceal their activities. Suggest that clients always draw curtains at night so that a potential intruder cannot see what they are doing or who is with them.

Persuade clients that anyone knocking on the door and requesting entry should be asked for proof of identity. Conmen are convincing liars and nearly always look plausible. Genuine callers doing surveys, repairing roofs, reading the meter, from the council or police will always be able to prove who they are. If in doubt, clients should ask the caller to return later while they ring the caller's office to check up on them. Warn clients if there is a spate of conmen in your area.

Some clients still distrust banks and post offices and hide their savings at home. You should do everything you can to discourage this, explaining that a fire or burglary could leave them with nothing. Try to persuade clients not to put a purse on top of a shopping bag nor to put a handbag down to one side while paying at tills. People collecting allowances should put the money away in a zipped bag, preferably a shoulder bag, before leaving the post office counter and should pay bills by Giro or cheque rather than in cash. Explain that the less cash clients carry with them the better.

A personal alarm which shrills loudly when activated may help increase a client's feeling of security when on the street, but emphasize to clients that an alarm is only useful if it is always at the ready and no good at all if it is at the bottom of a shopping trolley.

The best deterrent to street crime is to look confident, something many of your clients may find hard if they are not able-bodied, but tell them that physical frailty can be offset by keeping their heads up and looking around in an alert way. Encourage them to trust their instinct if they sense that something is wrong and to shout for help as loudly as possible if they feel in real danger. Most attackers and thieves are cowards looking for easy targets and melt away if faced with the challenge of an embarrassingly loud voice.

Coping with crime

There is no such place as a home that is truly burglar-proof, just as no one can guarantee that even the strongest and most confident-looking person will never be attacked. Sometimes crimes do occur. Tell your clients that their effects can often be made less serious and upsetting by trying some of these tactics:

- It is always worth trying to talk your way out of trouble – for instance, pretending that an intruder is in the house by mistake; ordering him to leave; pretending that someone else is in the house with you.
- Keep keys in the hand when approaching the house; that way you need not fumble on the doorstep and can gain entry quickly.
- If the key will not work the chances are an intruder is inside and has put down the lock on the inside; call the police immediately from a neighbour's house.
- Do not try to use a weapon on an attacker, the chances are he will snatch it away and use it on you.
- Give the police descriptions of any intruders actually seen; jot down any car numbers of vehicles that might have been involved.
- Trust your judgement; only you can sum up the situation.

Clients who have been victims of burglary and assault will be deeply upset, often feeling that both they and their homes have been permanently soiled by the crime or that they are to blame. They may need to cry, to tell the story over and over again and to express anger. Reassure them that it is normal to feel like this, but point out that what happened was not their fault and that they have survived the event, often by behaving bravely and cleverly in difficult circumstances. Clients will eventually recover their confidence, but such recovery is helped and speeded along enormously by two factors: the presence of a patient and sympathetic listener, and a total review of their security arrangements. New locks and bolts can have a very calming effect, especially if they are preceded by a visit from the local crime prevention officer. This useful police service is freely available and gladly given.

Summary

This chapter has emphasized the importance of safety-consciousness in carers and their clients in order to make the environment as free from hazards as possible.

The procedure for making 999 calls was outlined; this service should be used whenever in doubt, as the emergency services are expert at judging the seriousness of an incident. Special preventive measures against fire have been described, including the importance of providing ashtrays for smokers and discouraging smoking in bed, guarding open fires, taking precautions against chip pan fires and fires from faulty wiring or foam-filled furniture. Simple measures for dealing with fire were described, but the chapter emphasized the importance of leaving rescue to the fire brigade. The routine for dealing with a gas leak was described, again emphasizing the importance of carers putting their own safety first.

The section on medical emergencies stressed the importance of practical first-aid training. It gave guidelines on dealing with unconsciousness, choking, bleeding, shock, heart attack, burns and scalds, electric shock, poisoning, stroke, epileptic fits, hypothermia and falls.

The section on security passed on some basic advice on the importance of good-quality locks, bolts and doors and deterring street crime by taking care of money safely and looking confident. Where crimes do occur, there were some hints on how to minimize trouble and avoid violence. In the aftermath of crime carers often have a key role in arranging better security protection for clients and in comforting and reassuring them.

7

Death and bereavement

When you are dealing with a client group which contains many frail, vulnerable people, it is inevitable that your work will bring you into direct contact with dying people. You may have to comfort dying clients, deal with their distressed relatives, help other clients come to terms with the death of a friend or relation, help lay out the client's body, help make suitable administrative arrangements – for instance, contacting doctors and undertakers – as well as coming to terms with your own feelings. None of these processes is easy. The aim of this chapter is to pass on some of the ideas and ways of coping which others in this work have found useful.

Attitudes to death

Our society does not deal with death well. As the twentieth century has progressed, death has in many ways become an increasingly difficult topic. People speak of someone 'passing on', 'going', 'passing over', 'going to rest'. A person whose spouse or child has died is often described as having 'lost' them, as if they had merely been mislaid. In 1987, a television series about death eventually had to be called *Merely Mortal* because using the word 'death' in the title was thought likely to be off-putting to viewers. The words 'death', 'dead' and 'died' are generally avoided, as a way, perhaps, of avoiding its pain and mystery.

Why is this? One reason is that for most people, the death of someone close is a rare event. In the early years of the century this was not so. Children frequently died in infancy, young adults died of infections, and fewer people reached old age, so most people would have been far more familiar with death than is the case today when in many families there may be four or even five generations alive simultaneously. Also, in the past, most people died in their own homes, and their families would have nursed them through the closing stages of their lives. Today 60 per cent of all deaths take place in hospitals, so that most of us have never lived through the ebbing away of life in a loved one and many have never seen a dead body.

At the same time, almost all the rituals that used to be associated with death are disappearing. People no longer pause respectfully when a funeral procession passes in the street; blinds and curtains are not drawn in neighbours' houses. It is no longer considered essential to wear black or for women to wear hats to a funeral and the bereaved relatives are certainly not expected to wear black after it. There is no set period of mourning where the bereaved are allowed to express their grief through comforting rituals such as being visited by a constant stream of friends and family, wearing certain clothes and being allowed to cry. Non-churchgoers are not visited by ministers, religious services at funerals are beginning to disappear in a secular society, and the demand for non-religious funerals is growing. Some people are now arranging the cremation of their relatives, at the dead person's specific request, without a funeral service at all. Even at traditional funerals, there is quite often a request not to send flowers but to make a donation to a named charity instead.

All these trends make it difficult to deal with death. The rituals of the past had a purpose. They were comforting, they helped people express grief openly, they allowed other people to mourn with the bereaved and they gave people time to adjust before they were expected to be 'normal' again, as these older people comment:

> Wearing black clothes was good. It was a way of saying 'I've experienced a devastating loss, I can't wear bright colours. Black expresses my feelings which are also black.' I hate this modern way of pretending people haven't died and you can wear anything to their funerals.

> In my village, the funerals were magnificent and people paid into schemes to make sure they had a good one themselves. The church or chapel was packed and we sang good hymns. People looked after you and the minister visited daily. The Sunday after the funeral the whole family went to chapel together and there was a special prayer. It meant a lot to people.

> When a funeral procession passed, everything came to a stop. Men doffed their caps, everyone bowed their heads. Now the

posh cars rush past and no one takes any notice. I don't think that's right, it hurts the people in the family.

Viewing the body is another ritual which has all but disappeared, yet it was a helpful way for many people of accepting that the death had actually happened and was final, as this woman, now 85 and living in a residential home, comments:

> I don't like the way that death is hushed up here with the body hustled out in secret. I think it's far better to do what we did in the old days. The body was laid out and put in an open coffin in the front parlour. It was a mark of respect for friends, family and neighbours to visit and to view the deceased.

> When my father died in a pit accident, this is what happened: I saw him in his coffin and was just terribly relieved. I'd imagined him with his face expressing agony and his body mutilated. He wasn't, he just looked peacefully asleep. But it made me realize that he really was dead and wasn't coming back.

Where grieving relatives do not see the body, there is now some evidence to suggest that adjustment takes longer because the bereaved person may postpone the process of learning to live again. Sometimes they cling to the fantasy that the dead person is still alive. For instance, in one extreme case, the widow of a serviceman killed in a helicopter accident abroad was reported to be still describing herself as 'married' on official forms and believing that her husband was alive more than twenty years later, because his body had never been found.

Certain other social trends have also made it more difficult to cope with death. Advances in medicine have now made many serious diseases treatable; at the same time, the slowing of the ageing process and the stress placed on preventive health through diet and exercise have tended to create the idea, however illogical, that death can somehow be postponed for ever. So terminal illness is seen as a personal defeat by both care staff and by clients.

In other cultures, where religion is still important in everyday life, death is handled better. Hindus set aside ten days for mourning when friends and relations offer gifts and friendship to the bereaved. Muslims mourn for a month, Sikhs for ten days, Jews for seven days. In most of these mourning rituals, open grieving is encouraged and bereaved people are not expected to go straight back into appearing normal but will continue to be supported by a variety of comforting rituals for many months afterwards.

In our own culture, death is an embarrassment. Dying and bereaved people are avoided, typically with excuses such as 'I wouldn't want to upset them', which can normally be more honestly put as 'I wouldn't want to upset myself'.

As a carer, it is normally impossible to avoid contact with dying and death. It is important, therefore, to start by trying to understand how clients feel.

The dying client

Working with a dying client will demand every ounce of your courage, skill and sensitivity. Some clients may know that they are dying and may accept the fact calmly. Others may have asked not to be told if their illness is terminal, but may nevertheless have guessed correctly that it is. Some clients may be frightened of the pain that, often wrongly, they anticipate. Others may be worried about how their families will cope after their death.

There has been much research into the emotions of dying people and one of the most distinguished investigators in the field, Elizabeth Kubler-Ross, has described in *Living with Death and Dying*, the typical cycle of feelings as falling into several stages:

denial   Clients will not accept the truth about their illness; they go on believing that they will recover.

anger   Clients feel resentful that others will survive; they wonder why they were singled out to be ill and what they did to deserve it.

bargaining   The client bargains with God for survival – 'Please God, if you let me live, I'll never be selfish again'.

depression   Everything feels hopeless; the client often feels suicidal or withdraws from communication with everyone.

acceptance   Finally the client accepts that death is inevitable, may redraft a will, ask to see special friends and family to say goodbye, may ask for spiritual guidance, and feels at peace.

Other researchers and writers have described other types of reaction, but they all emphasise the same basic idea of a cycle which includes denial, anger and acceptance. Some clients may never pass the stage of denial, some may quickly reach acceptance, others go round the whole cycle several times. Something like this was observed by this home care assistant:

> Jane had always been very fit until she developed Hodgkin's disease. She refused at first to believe the diagnosis, saying that she just had swollen glands and the doctors didn't know what they were talking about. Then, when she was repeatedly told that it was true, she couldn't believe that she would die and kept saying that she would live to be a hundred and that she was planning to build an extension to her house and that she was damned if she was going to accept anything that stood in the way. I noticed then that she did start talking about the seriousness of her illness, but then she got very angry and blamed the doctors for the slowness of the diagnosis. She had two long hospital stays but insisted on coming home because she said the district nurse and her GP and I could look after her a lot better than 'those fools' in the hospital. It was clear that she didn't have long to live, but she said she was determined to live to the spring because she hadn't spent all that money on spring bulbs for nothing, and she did. By then she was in a wheelchair and had to be readmitted to hospital several times and suddenly she got very depressed and refused food and visitors and cried a lot. She would still flare up with anger occasionally and would say that she would outlive us all yet. She insisted on going home, and a Macmillan nurse was arranged for her. Whether this made the difference I don't know, but this nurse was a very special person and spent hours, it seemed, listening and talking and also got her pain under control. Within a few days she was saying things like 'I'm ready to die, you know'. She was by then very weak but was determined to die at home. She talked to me about her young daughters and about her marriage, which had ended by then. She didn't have any religious faith, but that didn't seem to bother her. She told me she hoped she'd live on in the memories of people who'd loved her. In the end it was a peaceful death, very dignified, very easy, with no pain because her pain had been so well controlled with drugs, but never so much that

she wasn't aware of what was going on. She left us all beautiful letters thanking us for our care; I'll never part with mine.

Helping dying clients

What can you, as a carer, do to help a dying client? It is important to encourage the client to express any physical pain that he or she feels. The section on counselling will have given you some ideas for ways of opening the conversation, so use them in this situation, too. For instance ask how the client is feeling, and then wait and listen carefully to the reply, preferably sitting down on the bed or in another chair so that you are at the same eye level. Make it clear to the client that it is all right to say that she is in pain or discomfort and that staff will be concerned to control the pain *before* it develops rather than afterwards.

This is important because fear of pain is one of the main worries of a dying client and any pain will be felt more acutely if the client is worried and upset. Reassure the client that there is always relief from pain and that medicines will be prescribed to control it. The approach to pain in dying clients is now to prevent it developing at all by constantly moving in advance of pain rather than running to catch up with it. Side-effects of pain-relieving drugs are also treated. This way of looking at the problem is largely due to the successful work of the hospice movement, which has developed an approach to terminally ill people which offers them a loving, calm and cheerful environment made possible by skilful pain control.

When pain-relieving drugs are prescribed and a client still reports pain to you, you should tell the appropriate senior person immediately so that the client's drugs can be changed or the dose altered.

Simply being with clients, holding their hands, if this is their wish, can in itself relieve pain because the client no longer feels so alone. The presence and touch of another human being is profoundly reassuring. Carers sometimes avoid dying clients because they cannot bear to see their distress, but this is a mistake, even though it may take courage to overcome such feelings. Dying clients, above all, need their self-esteem constantly reinforced. They may feel distressed by their gaunt appearance, by incontinence or by offensive odour from a cancer. To feel that they have also become untouchable at such a time is an extra and painful burden.

Here is how some carers approach this task:

> I never pass the room of a dying client without going in and I never go out again without touching the client. Sometimes I'll hold a hand, sometimes I just put the back of my hand on the client's forehead. Clients are used to nurses checking their pulse at the wrist, so they just accept that touch from us, too.
>
> I noticed some of my colleagues avoided eye contact with dying clients and never touched them. I felt that was awful, people need touch so much more at that time. I once sat for half an hour holding a client's hand and he clutched me so tightly . . .! As I got up to go I saw a tear start and he said 'thank you for holding my hand – I feel less like a leper now'.
>
> We are not supposed to leave doors open because of the fire risk, but when a client is dying, I prop the door open and always pause to say 'hello', and 'is there anything you need?'

Pressure sores can develop quickly in dying clients. These are sores which develop in bony parts of the body such as heels, elbow and hips as a result of lying too long in one position. They can quickly become deep and are extremely painful. The best treatment is prevention by regular turning of clients. Dying clients are particularly at risk of developing pressure sores as they may have become very thin and their illness may be keeping them immobile. Incontinence also increases the risk of pressure sores. Remembering to turn clients every few hours according to the plan set out for their care will be an important part of keeping them comfortable. Net beds, sheepskins and ripple mattresses will help, and so will special cushions designed to reduce rubbing.

You may be able to find other ways of keeping clients physically comfortable in their beds and chairs, for instance by making sure that they always have plenty of pillows, are offered a small neck pillow or one of the large triangular sort which supports the shoulders as well as the head. A bed cradle may be necessary to keep bed clothes from pressing painfully on feet and a cold compress can relieve headache. Keep bed linen fresh and clean, changing it frequently to help the client remain comfortable.

Other common problems are a dry, ulcerated mouth, constipation, haemorrhoids (piles) and cystitis (a painful bladder infection). Again, report these and help other staff carry out whatever measures are prescribed. For instance, a dry mouth, even in a client who cannot swallow, can be relieved by patting with some moistened gauze, or offering a small piece of lemon and an ice- lolly. A dry, cracked mouth can be relieved by a cream. Haemorrhoids can be treated with suppositories and cystitis with antibiotics.

Keep any routine procedures as gentle and brief as possible. So, for instance, it may be better to give a client a bed bath than to try to offer a full bath, if by doing so you tire the client less. When you are checking for pressure sores, combine this with turning and any other treatment, so that you disturb the client as little as possible. Any time you gain in this way will probably be far better spent talking to the client.

Remember that even apparently unconscious people may still be able to hear and understand, so never have conversations, even whispered ones, with colleagues or relatives in the client's room. Do so right out of earshot. At the same time, if you have to wash or turn an unconscious client, you should continue to speak to them as if they can hear, using their name and explaining what you are doing.

The look and feel of a client's room can make a real contribution to the sense of comfort and care that they feel in their last days of life. A hushed, dark cool atmosphere will not be helpful. On the other hand, it will help to have a softly lit, cheerful, warm environment which has flowers, plants, pictures and cards because they all suggest love, hope and the idea that there is more to life than mere existence.

Spiritual matters

The spiritual dimension is important. Terminal illness usually means that most clients want to try to make sense of their lives, to think about the meaning of it all, to grapple with the possibility of an afterlife and the unknown which lies ahead. Whether or not clients believe in God, or are members of a particular religion, these questions are likely to trouble them. Some clients may have a strong religious faith which deserts them at this testing time, some rediscover flagging faith, some find that their faith remains steady. One study showed that dying clients either with religious faith or with none were the most free from anxiety, and it was the waverers who had most problems in relation to spiritual issues. How should you handle this topic?

I don't belong to any formal religion myself, but I do ask clients if anyone checked whether or not they want to see our chaplain, or some other religious adviser. From the reaction to that, you can usually tell a lot. For instance, some clients are immediately hostile and say they can't bear religion, while others hesitate and look a bit interested, so I say something like 'How important is religion to you?' Often we get into a long conversation then. I think it definitely helps the clients and these conversations certainly help me because who doesn't ponder these things?

This woman works as a volunteer in a hospice, and finds that her own religious beliefs help her in approaching clients:

Everyone knows that this place is run by people who are practising Christians, but we have clients here from all religions. As a Christian, I'm not embarrassed to talk about religion and clients know this. I've often prayed with people just in an informal way. Sometimes we thank God for their lives, sometimes we just pray for enlightenment. A lot of people want to make confessions or have a sacrament arranged, so we always have priests and ministers available. But a lot of our clients don't have any formal religion at all – even so, they are often relieved to know that they can have 'spiritual' conversation if they want to.

If you work in a residential or hospital setting, clients will already have been asked to declare their religion. This is important in a multicultural society as each religion has its own practices and beliefs. Roman Catholics may want to celebrate various sacraments, including the Eucharist and the anointing of the sick ('extreme unction'). Other Christians may want various forms of 'healing ministry', sometimes described as the 'laying on of hands'. Jews may wish a rabbi to say prayers and to help them acknowledge their sins; Hindus may want to lie on the floor in a wish to be as near to 'mother earth' as possible. Muslim clients may try to continue their daily routine of prayer five times daily with each time of prayer preceded by washing face, hands and arms.

There are many other important aspects of religious rites which clients may wish to carry out, with or without family or with a priest or adviser. These will vary from one client and one religion to another, and it is important to ask clients if they have such needs and to help them come to terms with what it is actually possible for them to do.

You may also have the opportunity to encourage clients to make a will. As with so much else in this chapter, this is a sensitive topic. Avoiding making a will is a way of going on denying that death is imminent, and clients still focused on this stage of adjustment may never acknowledge the need to make their intentions clear. Many clients, however, will want to sort out their affairs, not least to prevent the troublesome quarrels and family resentments which can occur in the absence of a will. This home care assistant comments on the difficulties that can result from the absence of a will:

> I looked after a man who had allowed his house to get into a dreadful state because he just couldn't afford to repair it. It was a big house and was in a nice area, so it was worth a mint. Three of his four children had ignored him. His eldest daughter had been very good, visiting every other day. It was obvious he was dying, but he just couldn't accept it and no one, including me, was brave enough to say to him 'Now have you made a will?'. When he died, it was clear that he hadn't. His money was divided equally between the four children and the eldest daughter still doesn't speak to the other three; there's now a complete family split. I'm sure if he'd made his intentions clear, and who can say what they were, that at least could have been avoided.

The benefits to clients of making a will are very considerable, as these care assistants observe:

> It makes them feel that they can die with a clear conscience. There's a tremendous feeling of satisfaction; it helps with the adjustment to death because I always notice a sense of peace after the will has been signed and sealed.

> When you've got the right relationship with clients, you can talk about wills, whether they've made one, where it is, are they writing people letters as well, and so on. I think it's a wonderful thing to talk to clients about because it helps them see that they really do have a legacy to leave, not just material things, but spiritual and loving things as well.

You should avoid witnessing a will, but instead ask the client's solicitor to find witnesses. This is because it is possible that a will may be contested and it is better not to be drawn into such disputes. Where the client draws up a will while living in an institution, the will should be deposited in a safe place because it is an important document.

Some clients may also wish to donate organs for transplant or research. If so, make sure that these intentions are written up in their notes and records, as action needs to be taken swiftly after the client's death in order for organs to be useful.

The last hours of life

You need to be able to recognize the signs that a client may be in the last hours of life, as you may be the person in closest contact with the client. Relatives may need to be called. You may need to make extra effort to ensure that the client's death is in as peaceful and loving an environment as possible.

Some clients may die suddenly from a massive haemorrhage or thrombosis, but most will gradually become weaker and weaker, sinking imperceptibly into coma and then death. The signs that this is happening may include:

- mental and physical agitation, in spite of inability to express pain or discomfort in words because of physical weakness
- breathing becoming noisy and gasping, the pulse becoming weak and irregular
- refusing food or drink in spite of a very dry mouth
- facial expression becoming fixed with staring eyes which remain open even in unconsciousness
- incontinence, caused by muscle relaxation
- body temperature dropping, often including a cold sweat on face and hands.

Last offices

The phrase 'last offices' is used to describe the final services you offer a client after death but before burial or cremation. Depending on where you work, you may or may not have to take part in this final mark of respect for a client. For instance, if you work as a home care assistant, it is unlikely ever to be one of your duties, but if you work in a hospital or residential home, you may well be expected to take part.

You may find this prospect frightening if you have never done it before. However, a more positive way to look at 'laying out' a dead client is expressed by these two people, one a nursing auxiliary, the other a care assistant in a nursing home:

> I see it as much the same as the washing and caring I do for the live person; there's no difference really, is there?

> There is nothing ghoulish or frightening about a dead person. Often they look more peaceful and younger than they did in their last days of life. I also think it's nice for the relatives to know that the same person who looked after the client in life has looked after them in death.

Again, the actual procedures may be affected by the client's religion. For instance, the family of a Jewish client may wish to nominate a 'watcher', and the body may be washed by three people who form a 'burial society'. No cosmetics or embalming are allowed and the funeral must take place within twenty-four hours. The same time limit is imposed by Muslims, who also have washing and dressing rituals. For adherents of some Christian denominations it is considered important to put a rosary or crucifix in the dead client's hands. If you are not certain what religious restrictions there might be, you should consult your manager and the client's family immediately.

Where there are no religious rites to be followed, the usual procedure, usually begun about an hour after death, before rigor mortis (muscle contraction) sets in, is as follows:

- Drains and dressing are removed.
- The body is washed, and any wounds are redressed.
- An identity bracelet is left in place.
- Orifices are packed to avoid seepage.
- The body is redressed either in a shroud or normal clothes (some clients may have asked to be buried in a particular garment).
- Hair is brushed, nails trimmed and cleaned, male clients are shaved.
- Limbs are straightened, arms laid straight at sides.
- Dentures are normally left in but the mouth needs to be supported. Sometimes a bar of soap is tucked under the chin, sometimes a bandage is used.
- Jewellery is normally removed, but consult relatives about this; some people prefer a wedding ring, for instance, to be left in place.

- The bed is remade and the client's face is covered with a separate cloth.

Two people are needed to lay out a body because of the lifting involved and also because it is a task better shared than carried out alone. A quiet, purposeful atmosphere is essential, with the same respectful attitude shown to the client's privacy as when he or she was alive, so the body should not be exposed any more than is absolutely necessary during washing.

You should be aware that a dead person sometimes appears to breathe out but this is only the release of stored air and is quite normal.

Usually the room which contains the body is kept cool and dimly lit and may be decorated with flowers so that when relatives visit the room looks as little like a hospital room as possible.

In a residential home or hospital, you also need to be sensitive to the feelings of other clients. Your employers will have their own policy on these matters, but it is usually considered better not to remove a body secretly and in haste. Other clients will usually see this as offensive and upsetting, a foretaste of how *they* may in turn be treated, whisked away as if they were an embarrassment.

A better tactic is to tell other clients openly that so and so has died, to remove the body in an unhurried way to wherever it is to be laid out, and then to ask clients if they would like to see the dead person to pay their last respects.

Remember that with elderly clients, this is the custom they are likely to remember from their youth, and they may be grateful for the opportunity to say a formal goodbye to a friend.

The administrative procedures

These will vary from one employer to another, but certain basic procedures are normally followed to comply with the law. The senior member of staff present usually rings the client's doctor so that a death certificate can be issued in the case of an expected death. You should note the exact time of death and who was present. The undertaker is also contacted at this point, in consultation with the client's family.

If the death was unexpected, the doctor will certify that the client is dead, but may not issue a certificate. The police will be contacted and may wish to interview you or other staff about the circumstances.

The coroner's office has to give permission for the body to be moved to a mortuary before a post-mortem is carried out to find out the cause of death. There may have to be an inquest to establish this.

Helping relatives and friends

> When my mother was dying in a local home, both she and I had superb treatment. I was staggered by it all. They regarded me as being as much in need of their tender loving care as she was. That was such a help at a very difficult time.

This is as it should be; both clients and their families should be the focus of your attention. In practice, this may not be easy. You may feel furious at what you see as the neglect of clients by their families. Relatives themselves may be upset and hard to handle; you may find their visits intrusive. However, the solution to these difficulties is to be more, not less, involved with clients' families.

First, getting to know relatives can help you find out more about your clients, allowing you to care for them more fully. By the time they come into your care, clients may be seriously affected by physical or mental illness, and their ability to communicate their past lives and present preferences much diminished, as this care assistant comments:

> Talking to families of dying clients is really valuable. A person that you see as a very ill person has a whole history which you run the risk of not knowing unless someone can explain it to you or tell you about it. An elderly mentally infirm client who came to us terribly confused and in the terminal stages of his illness turned out to have been headmaster many years previously of my old school. You'd never have thought this poor, thin, wild figure could have done this job, but I began talking to him about the school and I swear he understood. Just for a few seconds he'd smile, and I knew I'd connected with him.

Relatives have a greater claim on the client than you and your colleagues. It is often difficult to see this clearly when you are involved for many hours daily with a client, but the client's family network is almost certainly far more complicated and deep-rooted in past and present emotion than you are able to perceive.

Understanding the relatives and getting to know them can also help head off the difficulties and misunderstandings which can arise when communication is limited, as in these cases:

> Mrs —— 's relatives insisted on visiting at funny times when fewer staff were on duty and after she died, they wrote a horrible letter saying she'd been badly treated. She hadn't at all, but we'd hardly ever spoken to them!

> There was a real mix-up about who counted as a next of kin. Both sons said they should have been informed before the daughter. Since none of them had ever even visited it was difficult to sort out; all we could go on was what the meagre notes said.

Helping the dying client's family

There is a lot you can do to help the visitors of a dying client:

- Welcome them warmly, greeting them by name.
- Offer them tea, coffee, biscuits or sandwiches. This simple reassuring ritual of hospitality can do a lot to make people feel comfortable.
- Make it clear, if you are working in an institution, that relatives can come and go at any time.
- Involve them in the client's care – for instance, encouraging them to report any pain, to give cold compresses if the client has a headache, and reassuring them that everything that can be done is being done.
- Ask them if they want to be with the client at the moment of death, and make sure that you know how to contact them quickly if necessary.
- Offer them an armchair or folding bed in the same or a neighbouring room.
- After the client has died, ask if they want to see the body and arrange for them to do so in a tactful and sensitive way.

Understanding how bereaved relatives feel

Where you are working with older people, you may be especially conscious that their loss may be a serious blow. The survivor in a long-lasting marriage will need to learn to manage alone after a lifetime of support. The loss of married status may be harshly felt and there is likely to be loss of income, too. Where the survivor is a son or daughter, the loss may be felt equally acutely, as this bereaved daughter comments:

> I looked after my mother for about fifteen years and was exhausted by the whole thing. I am not young myself and caring for her took all my commitment. When she died everyone kept telling me it was 'a happy release'. I think they meant it was a release for me, not for her. Actually it bowled me over. My whole purpose in life had suddenly disappeared, and even though logically I knew I'd have leisure, money and time for myself, emotionally I felt I'd lost my reason for existence.

You also need to be aware that sometimes the relationship has not been a positive or happy one and the death brings mixed feelings of confusion and guilt, as in this case, described by the home care assistant who helped the couple concerned:

> Mr — had had a car accident eight years previously in which he had been responsible for the death of another driver. At the time of the accident he had a woman with him with whom he was having an affair. The business of the prosecution revealed the affair to his wife, but before it could all come to court he had a serious stroke which left him paralysed and pretty helpless. His wife looked after him for all those years even though he was consistently bad tempered and vile to her while being utterly dependent on her care. Even before he died, she told me that she had prayed for his death. When he did die she was overcome with remorse and guilt because she felt, superstitiously, that she had hastened it. I felt I actually helped a lot to ease this by just listening to her and reassuring her that this could not possibly have been so.

Even where the relationship is less fraught, family and friends are still likely to experience the same stages of coping with the loss described earlier in this chapter (page 121) in relation to the client. They will feel grief in various stages: denial, anger, depression and then acceptance, or something like this. These emotions are likely to be acutely felt, and can be overwhelming. These carers describe some of the ways in which bereaved relatives and friends experienced the death of a client:

> Mrs — reported seeing and hearing her husband. She said she felt he was in the house, even six months later, and often talked to him as if he was still there.

> Miss B and Mrs S had been close friends in our home. For the first month after Miss B died, Mrs S could not be parted from her friend's shawl; she clung to it and sobbed if you even tried to rearrange it for her.

> William died of a massive heart attack which had been preceded by a lot of pain in his jaw and shoulders. His wife was constantly going to the doctor saying she had the same pain and believed she also had heart disease. Even though nothing could be found, she was not reassured.

> For the first few weeks, every time I visited to do shopping and so on, his wife would rage and cry, saying if only he hadn't smoked so much he'd still be alive and how it was his fault he was dead and how could he have left her like this.

> He kept saying over and over again that if only they hadn't gone out shopping that day, it wouldn't have happened because she wouldn't have fallen . . . he seemed to feel that he'd been a bad husband and that this had caused her death.

> I had to tell her doctor that I thought there was a real risk of suicide. She said she felt her life was pointless without her husband and that no one would miss her if she died.

These are common expressions of grief. You may also encounter anxiety, drinking more alcohol 'to deaden the pain', weight loss and withdrawal from the company of friends and family.

Adjusting to normal living can take a long time – it is rarely complete by six months and may take up to two years before the acute pain of loss is replaced by the quieter sadness of acceptance. Here is how one home care assistant described the process of grieving in one of her clients:

> I looked after an elderly couple where the husband had emphysema and the wife was severely disabled by arthritis. When he died she needed a lot of support. In the week before his funeral she seemed numb and didn't cry very much. She

kept saying that she couldn't take it in that he'd died. His room was kept exactly as it had been, no one was allowed even to touch his pills and his bed was made up as if he was going to climb back into it. After the funeral she suddenly started crying continuously and needed a lot of help because she was so angry and said she felt 'deserted'. She blamed his employer, whether rightly or not I don't know, for his illness and kept saying she would sue them. After about six weeks she calmed down and seemed to become very apathetic, said she didn't care whether she lived or died and could hardly bring herself to talk to me when I did her housework, whereas before she'd been a great chatterbox. Her shopping list went down to practically nothing because she wasn't eating.

Things began to get a bit better when she was given a kitten and she said to me, looking a bit guilty, that she'd always wanted a cat but her husband hadn't liked them.

Another turning point was getting a phone. That put her in touch with some old friends and, because of her mobility difficulties, the council was able to arrange transport to see them now and again. After about a year she told me that although she'd never stop missing her husband, and still thought about him every day, his death did not hurt in the way that it once had.

How carers can help bereaved relatives

You may find it easier to think that relatives will not want you 'intruding' on their grief. You may feel that if they cry in front of you, you will feel embarrassed, or get upset yourself. You may worry about whether you can cope with the responsibility of trying to help someone who is overwhelmed with grief, and wish that they would control their feelings. The difficulties are neatly summed up by Colin Murray-Parkes in his classic book, *Bereavement: Studies of Grief in Adult Life*:

> It is best to get conventional verbal expressions of sympathy over as quickly as possible and to speak from the heart or not at all . . . Pain is inevitable in such a case and cannot be avoided. It stems from the awareness of both parties that neither can give the other what he wants. The helper cannot bring back

the person who is dead and the bereaved person cannot gratify the helper by seeming helped. No wonder that both feel dissatisfied with the encounter.

Getting past these barriers is not easy, but it is possible. You should try to make it clear that it is all right to cry and to get upset. You can encourage the bereaved person to grieve openly, because this expression of grief will help the process of coming to terms with his loss. Whereas many people, including other members of the family, will avoid the bereaved person, you can make a point of being available to him, given the time-limits your work will place upon you.

The fact that you are outside the family may be a help here. Family members may compete with each other to display grief or may conceal their feelings; the bereaved person may need to talk to someone not involved in the same way.

Some bereaved people are frightened by the power of their emotions at this time and worry that they are losing their sanity. You can reassure them that such emotions are normal and that these feelings will eventually become less overwhelming. Do this sensitively. To tell a bereaved person that in time he will feel his loss less strongly may seem to him to imply that the dead person can easily be forgotten or replaced. Better to say: 'Everyone feels something like this . . . most people find that these frightening feelings fade after a bit, even though people never lose their sense of sadness at the loss.'

Do not be afraid to talk about the dead person in a straightforward way. Many bereaved people are hurt by the way others avoid mentioning the dead person's name because it seems to suggest that their lives and achievements were unimportant. Bringing them into the conversation in a warm and natural way can be a tremendous relief, as this widow comments:

> My home help was a marvel when Charles died. Everyone else went out of their way to avoid mentioning him. I knew why, they were afraid I'd break down, but it was horrible not being able to talk about it. She was wonderful. She'd make a point of remembering some of the funny things he'd said and done, or would say things like what a wonderful display there was in the garden and how that was a tribute to his skill. She was the only person I could talk about him with. Everyone else seemed set on pretending that he'd never lived, which was so hurtful.

Be especially alert at anniversaries and times of celebration. Christmas, New Year, birthdays, wedding anniversaries and the anniversary of the death are all potentially sad and difficult days, but they can also be turning points, marking the fact that a considerable time has passed and that the period of mourning must come to an end.

Where adjustment is slow and painful, you should report this to your manager. Further investigation may prove the need for more skilled and intensive help.

Your own feelings

You are unlikely to be able to rise above the feelings that a death produces, particularly if you were fond of the client and had invested a lot of personal energy in your care for that person. The death of someone you knew well brings home the inevitability of your own death, and few of us are totally reconciled to that. Dealing with the raw emotion of other people's grief is also demanding.

There are no simple solutions to these problems, but there are some helpful ways of approaching them. If the death of a client has made you feel that you are unprepared in any way for your own death, then it may help to make a will, especially if you have children and some modest property (say small savings and a house). A will can always be revised later if your circumstances change, but making it is a sensible first step to recognizing your own mortality. Far from making you feel that you have in some superstitious way 'hastened' your death, it is much more likely to give you the inner satisfaction of knowing that you have acted sensibly.

Discussing your feelings with other staff and expressing any grief or worry you feel will help you come to terms with difficult emotions; you will find that your reactions are likely to be similar to theirs. Sharing them makes them less intense and more bearable.

Many carers involved constantly in the care of dying people have found that it helps to learn more by increasing their knowledge of the whole process, physical and mental. Some suggestions for further reading are given at the end of this book; your employer may also be able to send you on special training courses where you can learn special care techniques.

It will also help to realize that your own reactions to the death of a client of whom you were fond are likely to follow the pattern already described in this chapter. You yourself may experience a sense of disbelief that the death has happened, or guilt and worry that you might have done more, or in some sense prevented the death; you may feel anger with colleagues or with the system for appearing responsible for the client's death and an acute sense of loss before you enter the stage of calmer acceptance and a realization that you can adjust. Knowing that this is normal will undoubtedly help shorten the pain and make adjustment easier in the long term.

Summary

This chapter has explored the carer's work in relation to death and bereavement. Among the topics discussed are our society's reluctance to face up openly to the facts of death and the resulting difficulties for clients, relatives and carers in adjusting to death and dying.

Dying clients may pass through a cycle of adjustment which may include denial, anger and guilt, 'bargaining' as a way of putting off acceptance, depression and withdrawal from contact with others, and finally a peaceful acceptance that death is near.

Caring for dying clients involves an emphasis on their physical care, most importantly on the prevention of pain; on their emotional care, especially conveying to them that they are not alone and on allowing them to express their feelings. Their spiritual care will involve arranging access to religious advisers and helping them follow the religious rituals appropriate to their culture and views.

The last hours of life are usually marked by pronounced changes in breathing, skin, body temperature and facial expression; carers need to be alert to these. When a client dies, the procedure of 'laying out', usually described as 'last offices', is an extension of the care offered the living client and involves washing the body respectfully and preparing it for viewing by relatives and then for burial or cremation.

Helping relatives and friends come to terms with their loss is an important aspect of many carers' work, in spite of the difficulties this may pose. Again, grieving may follow a cycle which includes denial, anger and then a final acceptance which involves adjustment to a new life. Being sensitive to the feelings of loss that families and friends may experience and encouraging them to express their grief and talk about the dead person may help people through this difficult time.

Finally, carers need to be alert to their own needs when clients die, treating themselves kindly and taking every opportunity to express feelings to colleagues.

8

Looking after yourself

There is no doubt that caring is a stressful job. It is always physically tiring and is frequently mentally draining because, to do it well, you are always giving and not often receiving. This chapter is about how to keep the stress of the job under control.

What is stress?

Stress is what we experience when pressure gets out of control. Some pressure in life is essential; the secret is to have just the right amount. If you have too little, you experience boredom and feelings of use-lessness. You may feel perpetually tired even though you are not working hard. If you have too much pressure you are likely to feel constantly exhausted and irritable, and to feel that life generally is getting on top of you.

A life where stress is under control does not mean a life without pressure because that would mean a life without challenge, stimulus and the opportunity to grow and develop as a human being. Even so, finding the happy medium can be difficult. One reason for this is that what you experience as intolerably stressful might be an enjoyable challenge to a colleague; what another colleague finds boring, undemanding, and therefore stressful can be a pleasant routine to you. It is also important to remember that your own views on these topics will change as you become more experienced in the job. Looking back on your own first few weeks in any new job, you can probably remember aspects of it which you found stressful and difficult but which no longer cause you any difficulty.

Whatever the events or problems that trigger stress for you, the range of symptoms is normally the same for everyone. These all involve a change from what is normal for you and may include changes in your:

- sleep patterns
- eating patterns
- alcohol, tea or coffee drinking – usually more
- smoking – usually more
- mood – usually weepiness, irritability
- sexual behaviour – usually loss of interest in sex
- other behaviour – for instance, arriving at work late; wearing a grubby uniform; being more prone to accidents; losing concentration; being indecisive.

Stress is uncomfortable and can make you more prone to illness, perhaps because of the behaviour changes just listed as symptoms. If you drink and smoke more, sleep less and drive carelessly, your chances of illness and accident obviously increase. Even so, the most likely immediate effects are on your mental rather than your physical health. Contrary to popular myth, stress is probably not a prime cause of heart disease. However, because it causes anxiety and unhappiness it can affect all the important relationships in your life, so for this reason alone it is worth thinking about how to reduce it.

Why is caring stressful?

Any job is stressful when there is a combination of high demands, high constraints and low support. Caring is a classic case. As a carer you probably make very high demands of yourself, and your organization may do the same. The constraints of the job are also considerable. For instance, the public expects a high standard of care; you may not be allowed a great deal of freedom in the way you carry out your job, and at the same time you may get very little support, perhaps in the form of training, from your manager. You may also not always be supported by your partner at home.

This section looks at some of the ways in which the caring environment can, wittingly or unwittingly, encourage the growth of stress.

The clients

One of the main reasons why caring is stressful is that you are dealing with such a vulnerable group of people. Seeing their distress, experiencing their problems at close quarters, will inevitably affect you. Here is a home carer whose case load includes a high percentage of clients with Alzheimer's disease (senile dementia).

> They can't help it, poor things, but their illness produces such bizarre behaviour. It's awful for them when they are still well enough to understand, however dimly, what is going on. Even worse than that, though, is to experience the terrible effects on their relatives. The pain and strain of living with a demented person day in, day out, is dreadful. Very very often, the husband or wife of such clients breaks down and cries on me. The effort of staying calm and not crying with them costs me such a lot!

A further problem is that it may be difficult to communicate with clients; they may have had physical or mental handicaps from birth, there may be language problems because English is not their mother tongue; or physical illness in adult life may produce conditions which create communication problems. Whatever the cause, the effects are similar – clients who cannot readily understand or communicate with you. This carer working with elderly confused clients, comments on the stress it can cause:

> It's very hard. I can sometimes say about twenty times, 'Please don't do that', or 'Bring the plate to me', and it's just as if I've never said it. It makes you feel like screaming, but of course there's no point in screaming, is there?

These problems of communication are taxing to carers because they appear to take away from you one of the main rewards of caring, which is knowing *from clients themselves* that they value what you do. If clients cannot tell you, or are not even able to register that they have noticed your efforts, this makes the job of caring much more stressful.

Then, too, there is the likelihood that for many of your clients there is no prospect of them getting better. Many of us like to feel that all illness is curable, and that recovery is an achievable goal. For many carers the reverse is true; their clients cannot get better, they can only get worse. Again, this can be hard to bear, especially where you have become fond of a particular client, as is the case for this warden of a sheltered housing scheme:

Our clients stay a long time because they are all more or less able-bodied when they move in. They tend to be interesting, alert and intelligent people and they can be very entertaining company, so you get fond of them. It's very very sad, and I do try not to let it affect me, but of course it does, if they succumb to the sort of illness where you have to see them slowly fading away, and you know that there's absolutely nothing anyone can do. I still feel a sense of personal loss and pain about one client whom I saw every day and who always had a laugh and a joke with me. He contracted leukaemia and took a long time dying. It was heartbreaking.

Where a lot of your clients are elderly, it is inevitable that many of them will die. Death is still a difficult topic for many of us, and ordinary experience does not prepare us for coping with the reality of it; hence the stress you may feel when the death of clients is frequently part of your experience of work. (The chapter on death and bereavement gives help on how to cope.)

With some clients, the problem is different: their behaviour is unpleasant and upsetting. Some clients are simply demanding, constantly creating little dramas and scenes designed to attract your attention. Others may take this behaviour further and may become offensive and rude; they may try to subject you to racial or sexual abuse.

A minority of clients may present even more extreme problems, where verbal abuse tips over into physical violence. This may be a common problem if your work involves dealing with people who have become drug-dependent, for instance on alcohol or heroin, or who suffer from physical conditions such as Huntington's chorea or Alzheimer's disease, where aggressive and violent behaviour can be one of the effects of their condition. Whatever the cause, working with such clients is stressful, as this regular volunteer at a night shelter scheme describes:

We set very clear rules about what is acceptable behaviour, but even so, you can *never* relax. You have to have eyes in the back of your head, looking out for bottles being smuggled in, fights developing that must be stopped at once, maintaining the kind of calm, friendly behaviour yourself that you want to encourage in clients . . . you finish your shift utterly knackered as a result.

Finally, working as a carer can be physically hard as well as mentally demanding. If you work in an institution you may be on your feet all day; if you work as a home care assistant, you may have to travel quite long distances to and from clients. Much of the work involves lifting; almost all of it involves standing for most of the day. No wonder carers get tired.

The job

When work is stressful, the cause often lies in the way the job is 'designed' – the features it has, or lacks, which tend to make us feel that the job is worth doing or not. Research has shown that whatever the job, there are certain things that make for good job design. A well-designed job will:

- be worthwhile – you and others will feel that it is important
- give you control over what you do – for instance, allow you to make decisions about whom you see, how much time you spend with them, how you deal with them and so on
- give you the resources you need to do it well – for instance, well-maintained equipment or a big enough budget
- make sure that you have the knowledge and skill you need, perhaps by training you
- make sure that you have 'feedback' on your work – for instance encouraging your boss to comment on your work regularly and not just at an annual appraisal, and also by encouraging clients to tell you what they think of your work
- give you chances to grow and develop, for instance by preparing you for promotion
- make sure that you feel you are rewarded fairly for the work you do – financially or in other ways.

Only you can decide how well your own job scores in these respects. Also, only you can put these features in order of importance for you. For some people, good pay may have to be their first priority, with everything else taking a back seat. Others may attach more importance to knowing that what they do is valued by clients, however poor the pay. It may be worth your going through the list above and ticking the features you feel your present job has, as a way of pinpointing the problem areas, if any.

However, for many carers, the stress-creating parts of the way their jobs are designed focus on three particular areas: status, pay and resources. In spite of the critical importance of caring as a profession, many carers feel that their work is undervalued – not by clients and their families, but by the public at large:

> When you say you're a care assistant, people tend to go 'oh yes', in a way that suggests they think it's a job anyone could do.

Linked with this, and perhaps its cause, is low pay:

> We're at the bottom of the local government heap as far as pay goes. It really riles me. Everyone depends on us – management, clients and their relatives, yet no one will pay us proper money for doing this work that they all agree is vital.

If this feeling of being exploited is linked with underfunding for equipment and other resources, then the potential for stress is very considerable.

Yourself

Some of the stress you experience in caring work may not be caused by the job or the clients. It may occur because of your own personality or circumstances. For instance, if you have a full-time job and are also the single parent of several young children, then, whatever the job, there is considerable potential for stress in your life. If you are the kind of person who sets herself very high standards, at work and at home, then your life is likely to be stressful, because human beings find such perfection impossible.

Another important area of potential stress is the difficulty many carers have in being assertive: expressing their needs and speaking up, avoiding the trap either of being aggressive or of being passive and saying nothing.

> My boss treats me like a five-year-old. I boil inside but outwardly I just say meekly 'yes, certainly'. I really despise myself for doing it. Why can't I speak up?'
>
> I'm often asked to work overtime when I don't want to. I wish I had the knack of saying 'no' properly. I've been told off in the past for being rude.

Some of our clients are aggressive. Often it's not their fault. Even so, I find it difficult not to shout back. I'm afraid I often do, then I feel very ashamed afterwards, it's not really professional behaviour to behave as badly as they do, is it?

Keeping stress under control

Only you can find and develop the ways of coping with stress that work for you. Even so, this section gives you a 'menu' of ideas, gathered from other people's experience as carers, that may help.

Looking after yourself physically

The clothes you wear to work are important. The wrong ones can adversely affect your well-being and effectiveness in your job. If you have to wear a uniform, make sure that it is not too tight and gives you room to wear warm clothes underneath on cold days and allows you plenty of air on hot ones. Choose flat, flexible, well-fitting shoes with plenty of heel and arch support. Shoes that lace up fit better than the slip-on sort – an important consideration when you are on your feet all day long.

Back damage is extremely common among people in the caring professions. One of the reasons is that the spines of human beings are still designed as if we were four-legged animals. Being bipeds puts a lot of strain on the spine anyway. Lifting heavy weights puts it in even more danger of damage. Clients are heavy, mattresses are heavy, beds are heavy. When you have to move them, make sure you always follow this simple rule: stand as close as you can, bend from the knees (never from the hips), and keep your back straight. Some people find this easier to remember as 'SBS' – Stand close, Bend the knees, Straight spine.

As well as being careful with lifting, you also need to make sure that you do not put yourself at risk in other ways. Do not, for instance, agree to replace lightbulbs or take down curtains for cleaning if all you can stand on is a rickety old chair. If your employer or client does not have a good pair of steps, you should explain that you cannot do the job that day. Perhaps you, your client or employer could arrange to buy or borrow the steps so as to make such tasks easy and safe.

I'm often asked to do dangerous things and I fell once, sprained my ankle badly and was off work for a week . . . so never again! *But*, you've got to say 'no' nicely, otherwise next thing you know the client will be trying to sprint up the terrible old shaky steps on his own then bang, crash – an accident! So now what I say is, look I'm going to be no good to you if I fall off those terrible old steps, nor you to me if you do the same. I'll come in tomorrow and borrow Mrs — 's pair and do it for you then and you promise me you'll not try it on your own!

One of the ways that many of us try to forget the stresses in our lives is to turn for solace to alcohol, tobacco, or tranquillizers. Alcohol appears to offer release from cares and worries because it affects the part of the brain that controls our inhibitions. The nicotine in cigarettes is a stimulant; if you are a smoker, you may feel that you 'deserve' a cigarette (the same may be true if you enjoy drinking alcohol) as a reward for your hard day's work. This is particularly true for women. Research has shown that, for many women, having a cigarette is one of the few ways in which they feel they have any personal time when no one is making demands on them. Tranquillizers affect the part of the brain that produces feelings of anxiety. By temporarily suppressing these feelings, they appear to keep the anxiety under control.

The problem with all these substances is that they only disguise the stress temporarily by damping down the symptoms. They cannot cure the stress. Indeed, if you smoke or drink a lot regularly or come to depend on tranquillizers, you simply develop a fresh set of problems, not least the feelings of self-dislike which are produced by such dependency:

I started having a glass of wine when I finished my shift. I was dealing with very severely handicapped people in one of the old 'subnormality' hospitals and it was exhausting work, physically and mentally. You felt such pity for the patients, and you couldn't hope to see any of them get better, the way the place was run. After a bit, one glass of wine became two, then three. Many evenings I was falling asleep on the settee then waking up cold and feeling horrible at midnight. It was affecting my work, I was often hung over and I loathed myself for 'needing' the booze. It got to the point where I nearly let a patient drown in a bath because I was so hung over I couldn't concentrate. That shook me. I realized I had to look at the whole way I was managing myself. The frightening thing was that I wasn't actually drinking a huge amount, I was well within the so-called safe limits, yet I knew that alcohol really had a hold on me. I decided to give it up totally for six months, just to prove that I could. This was surprisingly easy. After six months I found I'd lost my taste for it, I suppose the real reason was that I'd compensated for the alcohol by doing other things, most notably taking up swimming. This really kept my stress under control, so I didn't need the alcohol!

When you feel that stress has made you over-dependent on alcohol, cigarettes or tranquillizers it is best to try to get to the cause of the stress first. If dependency is still a problem that you feel you cannot tackle on your own, then look for help; books and tapes are often a useful first step; failing that, look for a self-help group. Many GPs run 'giving up smoking' or 'cutting down on drink' groups. The support of other people often succeeds where solo efforts fail.

As the account above shows, exercise is often an effective distractor, as well as being vital for health. You may feel that you are so physically exhausted by your day that exercise would tire you out. Yet the striking fact about exercise is that it actually refreshes you and gives you more energy. The adrenalin you produce is also an excellent way of discharging pent-up feelings. Here is a care officer, working in a hostel, describing why she plays badminton twice a week:

All my aggressive instincts go into thwacking that shuttle. It's 'take *that* Mr ——' and 'see if I care about *that*' as I hit it. I only play singles badminton because doubles isn't violent enough! By the time I've played for an hour, I'm totally relaxed; tired, but in a good way. If for some reason I can't play, I feel the stress mounting up and I get to screaming point at work much more quickly.

Brisk exercise – walking, swimming, jogging, or a racquet sport – for about thirty minutes three times a week is probably enough to keep the stress gremlins at bay as well as being the right amount to help keep your heart healthy.

When you are feeling stressed, you may find that your appetite is affected; perhaps you find it easier to resort to junk food because it is quick to cook and eat. Perhaps you skip meals altogether. To look after yourself properly it is important to be as careful about your own diet as you are about your clients'. Stick to the rules of modern healthy eating – raw, fresh fruit and vegetables whenever possible, wholemeal bread, rice and pasta, fish and white meat, with the minimum of fat, sugar and salt. A diet along these lines will help keep you at the weight that is right for you as well as making you feel energetic and vigorous.

Learning to relax

Many people find that it is helpful to learn a relaxation technique. There are many variants on the same theme; all essentially involve learning to breathe correctly from the diaphragm rather than the upper chest, then to relax one group of muscles at a time until your whole body is soft and floppy. Along with this muscular relaxation, you learn how to empty your mind of all the distractions and worries which will keep the cycle of stress and tension going unless you learn to stop it. To use these relaxation techniques successfully you need

- a quiet room where you will not be disturbed
- to lie down and close your eyes
- a friend to 'talk you down' or a self-teaching relaxation tape of the type sold in most 'health food' shops and bookshops
- plenty of time – at least thirty minutes.

Once you have successfully learnt the techniques of relaxation, you should be able to use them at any time to 'recharge'. Many people claim that half an hour of deep and deliberate relaxation is worth several hours of actual sleep because of the feelings of both tranquillity and energy it can produce.

Learn assertiveness

Much of the frustration and therefore much of the stress of a caring job is that you can feel powerless in relation to the other people, including the clients, in your life. Feeling that you have no control over your work is a classic recipe for job stress. Research has shown again and again that the popular idea of the over-stressed chief executive is a myth. The chief executive enjoys his life because he has power and choice. It is his lower-paid workforce who are likely to suffer from stress, especially if they are working on a production line where they cannot even control the pace of their work, let alone its content.

One way to increase the sense of control and power you have at work is to learn to be assertive. Assertiveness means that you state your needs clearly and calmly. It does not mean being aggressive; aggressiveness means stating your needs rudely and without consideration for others and is just as inappropriate as being passive and not stating your needs at all.

Assertiveness means behaving straightforwardly and honestly, avoiding the traps of behaving like a martyr ('I'm the only person round here who really cares about clients') or always blaming other people for events and feelings that are really your responsibility. It means refusing to take responsibility for things that rightly belong to someone else. Assertiveness means that you are willing to speak up for yourself, to say 'yes' or 'no' for yourself, to make mistakes and to ask for what you want – even if this does not guarantee that you will get it.

Assertiveness is different from both aggressiveness and passivity. For instance, a colleague asks you if you would toilet three clients. You already have six clients of your own to deal with and do not feel you can take on the additional work.

The *aggressive* response would be to say something like 'Of course I can't – I'm far too busy, can't you see that?'. This is likely to upset your colleague and to earn you a reputation for being difficult.

The *passive* response would be to say 'Oh well, all right then, I suppose I can'. This time you are likely to feel resentful and angry inside.

The only response that leaves you with self-respect and the respect of colleagues is the *assertive* one where you say in a friendly, calm way: 'No I can't really do it because I've got my own six clients to toilet, sorry. Is there someone else you could ask?'

Assertiveness means being able to

- *Say 'no'* to unreasonable requests, or even to reasonable ones if you do not want to say 'yes' without elaborate apologizing and excuses, so for instance, you could refuse to do overtime:

  We are very understaffed here so we are constantly asked to work extra time. I sympathize, but if I don't want the extra work I explain that I can't do it.

- *Admit your mistakes*
  Everyone is entitled to make mistakes; perfection is impossible. Rather than covering them up, assertiveness makes it possible to admit to them candidly, asking for help if necessary to avoid making them in future. For example:

  > I'm afraid I was a bit clumsy turning Mrs — this afternoon. I think I need you to show me again how to do that lift.

- *Speak up at meetings*
  It is often stressful to be at staff meetings where you want to speak up, but shyness or your worries about making a good impression hold you back. Staff meeting are occasions where you can share worries and ideas about the job and about clients with other people doing the same work. Here are some ideas about how to behave assertively at staff meetings:

  > I speak early in the meeting, the longer you put it off, the harder it gets.

  > I remember that other people are nervous, too.

  > I raise my doubts about things, often you find that other people share them.

  > I join in everything, but I aim to keep it brief, just a sentence or two.

- *Express dissatisfaction with the job to your boss*
  Voicing your worries and dissatisfactions is an important way of controlling stress. Tell your boss rather than keeping it to yourself:

  > I felt that we used far too much physical restraint on clients; things like seat belts and harnesses, or keeping them in cots all day long. It was causing me stress because it went against my principles. In the end I raised it with my boss. She seemed a bit surprised and said that it was for the clients' own good and how else could we cope with so few staff? I suggested that we were being asked to do these things as a way of disguising staff shortages, so she ought to raise it with *her* boss. It won't change overnight, but we've started a discussion, at least.

- *Ask for what you want*
  Many carers leave the work, even though they like it, because they cannot bring themselves to ask for some of the things

that would make their lives easier – extra equipment, promotion, different ways of organizing the work, and so on.

Many people, especially women, find assertiveness difficult because we tend to have been trained from our earliest days to put the needs of others first. This can make it very difficult to say 'no', to ask for things, or even to accept compliments. Assertive behaviour does not guarantee that you will always get what you want, but it is a useful tool for increasing self-respect and can often be an immensely powerful way of increasing the respect of others:

> I did a course on assertiveness, and I can honestly say that it has changed my life. I no longer feel put upon by either my family or my boss. I work in a half-way house, and it's very intensive, very stressful, working with clients who are leaving hospitals and getting back into the community. Some of them are very manipulative and I find I can now confront them openly. I've also been able to go to my boss and ask to have my grade and salary reviewed (I don't know yet if this will have a happy ending – but at least I've asked instead of sitting and stewing about it!) and I've asked for special training, which I'm getting, on alcohol and solvent abuse. I'd never have done any of this if I hadn't realized how important it is to be assertive.

Keeping your distance

One of the traps of caring as a job is of becoming over-involved with clients. If you allow this to happen, you are at grave risk of increasing the stress levels in your work. Once you allow a client to become more like a friend, you take on additional responsibilities and potentially additional worries. As a carer you are a professional. This means always remembering that you are paid to stay aware of the boundary between yourself and your client. You are not in their lives as a friend. Remembering this will help keep stress levels down, and will also prevent the misunderstandings and complications that can develop from over-involvement. Here is one such cautionary tale from a home care assistant who let the boundary become blurred:

> I first met Charles when he came out of hospital after a cancer operation. We got on well from the start and soon discovered that we were both committed Christians. I suggested that he

joined my family at our local church on Sundays and that led to his coming regularly to Sunday lunch. I felt very sorry for him because his wife had died and his son had emigrated, so he had no one at all for company. Eventually he had to have another series of operations and I couldn't bear the thought of his going home alone, so I invited him to stay with us. We had to curtain off our dining area and put a bed in it for him. It was obvious he didn't have very long to live. In fact a few weeks later he went back to hospital and died there. In his will, to our great surprise he left me his car, which was almost new. There was a tremendous fuss, his son wanted to contest the will, my bosses got involved – it was awful. In the end I kept the car, but the whole thing was horrible.

This carer's mistake was to invite her client into her private life. The client became over-dependent on her (and perhaps she on him) which laid her open to accusations, however unjust, of misconduct. Keeping some barriers in place is safer in the long run.

Talk it through with others

One of the simplest and most effective remedies for stress is to unburden yourself to a colleague, partner or friend. Keeping your worries bottled up is one of the surest ways to let them grow and flourish. Choose someone who is a good listener, along the lines discussed in Chapter 5, and let them help you. There is no shame in seeking help in this way. Indeed many groups of people in the 'caring professions' now make provision for colleagues to be able to share worries and thus unburden themselves of some of the stresses of the work.

Finally, accept that perfection in caring work is impossible. Set high standards, by all means, but forgive yourself generously when you fall below them.

Summary

Pressure and stress are not the same; stress occurs when pressure grows out of control. The secret of stress control is to keep the pressure at the right level. Caring can be stressful because the clients themselves demand a level of emotional commitment from their carers because of their physical or mental vulnerability or because of behaviour problems. The work is also physically tiring and often badly paid. The solutions to keeping stress under control might include:

- taking care to wear comfortable clothing
- learning to lift correctly
- keeping physically fit
- learning relaxation techniques
- learning to be assertive and to ask for what you want
- forgiving yourself for failure.

9

Making progress

As a care worker, you are likely to have acquired experience and skills which will be highly relevant to other jobs and attractive to other employers. For instance, you will have learnt how to cope with life and death emergencies, keeping a cool head as well as acting appropriately. You will have learnt how to listen effectively and how to help other people sort out difficult problems without butting in with your own views and opinions. You will have acquired a client-conscious attitude which helps frail people keep their independence and self-esteem even when they are dependent on others for help with daily living.

Improving the way you do your present job

Doing a job well is usually a source of pride and increases the satisfaction that you feel in your work. Since caring work is always taxing and it is hard to feel that you do it perfectly, there are usually ways to improve.

In a well-run organization, the employer will help you do this, normally by

- agreeing targets with you every twelve months
- linking the reaching of these targets with your pay and promotion
- giving you the opportunity at an 'appraisal interview' where your performance is reviewed, to say how you feel about the job and your bosses
- inviting you to identify areas of your work where you feel you could benefit from training.

Where they are well run, these schemes help both you and your employer. For you, it gives you feedback from the employer on how you and your work are viewed, so where things are going well, it is a tremendous boost to morale. It can also give opportunities to concentrate on the areas of weakness, where, with a little help from other staff or from training, you can improve the quality of your work.

If your employer runs this type of appraisal scheme, you should take every advantage of it. Do not be afraid to speak up and to protest if you think your targets are unrealistic or even not demanding enough. All such schemes give you an opportunity to declare your interest in 'personal development', and this is the time to state that you feel you want to be considered for promotion or to receive training in some particular aspect of the job.

Even if your employer does not offer you an appraisal system, and many do not, then you can still benefit from the ideas behind such schemes. On a piece of paper, jot down answers to these questions:

The past six months
- What achievements am I specially proud of?
- What aspects of my work do I need to improve?

The future
- What are my main work goals for the next six months?
- What will help me achieve them?
- What might stand in my way?

Having done this, you may come to the conclusion that you need further training. There are various ways, informal and formal, that you can do this. One of the easiest and most effective is simply to ask your immediate boss to give you more supervision and comment on your work. This is normally called 'coaching' and has a slightly different meaning from its popular use, where it often implies the intensive cramming of a school child for a public examination. In work terms, it means that your manager promises to take a planned and deliberate interest in your performance, offering you frequent help through friendly, constructive criticism. You may be lucky enough to have a boss who does this anyway, but experience suggests that after the first few weeks in a job, most managers stop offering a new employee any criticism, and real 'coaching' is surprisingly rare.

As well as on-the-job coaching, you should take every opportunity to look for short training courses in particular subjects. These may vary in length: one- and two-day courses are probably the most common, but other courses may last a week or even two weeks.

Typically, such courses may be on aspects of continence, on helping clients overcoming physical disabilities, on dealing with violence and aggression, or on 'reality orientation' for the elderly mentally infirm. Longer courses are normally linked with qualifications, and are run by local colleges of further education on a one-day-a-week basis over a year where your employer pays the fees (though many individuals also pay for themselves).

The advantages of longer courses are considerable. First, you learn more. Second, you meet other people in similar work but from different workplaces. This is valuable as a way of consolidating your own experience and of challenging yourself with different opinions. Then, of course, you also acquire a qualification, one of the main passports to more confidence, to promotion or to a complete change of career.

Looking to your future

Working as a care assistant, care officer or home care assistant may suit both your present and your future circumstances, as the work is interesting and undoubtedly socially valuable. However, it is certainly not well paid.

In future, you may want or need to improve your salary, and to progress to a more senior job. There are many possibilities where your present work will be seen as a considerable asset: proof that you have experience and skill relevant to a wide range of other occupations. Some of the main areas of possible progression are listed here.

Care management

The simplest way to progress is to look for promotion into a supervisory or management role within your present type of work. If you do not already know the answer, ask your present boss how she came to her job and what experience and qualifications she has. This will give you some idea of how your own experience and qualifications match up, and how you might look to fill any gaps, through more experience or further training.

You will already know that there is a thriving private sector in care work which is set to expand, partly as a result of government policy, and partly because of the predicted growth in the numbers of people needing care. Many privately owned residential homes are run by former care assistants who had one of the best possible pre-parations for running their own homes – being employed by other people in the same work. What such work will not necessarily have prepared you for is the business aspects. Running a home, or some other care service, means running a business.

Training and information can help enormously in making sure you do not fall into the commonest traps. Most of the major banks have helpful free information packs for people thinking of starting their own business (after all, it is very much in the bank's interest for your venture to be a success). Many other short courses, often sponsored by government departments, are run through local colleges and universities. They are either free or offered at very reasonable rates. Look in your local paper or ask at the job centre for details.

Nursing and allied fields

There is a crisis in nurse recruitment because the drop in the number of teenagers has coincided with a rise in demand for medical services of all kinds as well as the greater expectations we all tend to have of a higher-quality service when we do fall ill. Falling morale in the NHS and the expansion of opportunities in other careers have reduced the percentage of eighteen-year-olds who do opt for nursing. A major reorganization of nursing training, Project 2000, is also creating demand for more staff because more nursing training will be done in colleges and less on the wards.

As a result, there are now many areas of nursing and other professions in the care field where it is being made progressively easier to enter as a mature recruit. The opportunities include the nursing staff needed to keep a modern hospital in business, as well as all the important support staff – for instance, the people who fit wigs for cancer patients who have lost their own hair as a result of chemotherapy, the ambulance staff who provide transport for frail patients as well as first-line treatment for emergencies, the physio-therapists, occupational and speech therapists whose role is to hasten recovery – all these are fields where the demand for new staff will continue to grow and where there is the same client-conscious approach as you need for your current work.

For information on opportunities and training in these fields, contact your job centre. All job centres can now put you in touch with specialist employment advisers who will have up-to-date information on both national and local trends and who can advise on training. For queries relating specifically to nursing contact the National Board of Nursing in England, Wales, Scotland or Northern Ireland, according to where you live. Addresses on page 162.

Social work

Like nursing, social work is a rewarding job for those who can put clients and their needs first – one of the basic pillars of your present job. It encompasses a wide variety of jobs: the probation officer, the hostel warden, the nursing assistant working with young children, the instructor in day centres for adults with mental handicap, the person who deals with welfare rights, these are all examples of social work. The majority of these jobs are offered by local authorities, but many are also available in voluntary bodies or the private sector.

For some of the more junior jobs it is possible to enter without a qualification, as employers will provide training on the job. Increasingly, though, qualifications are being seen as essential for junior as well as senior jobs, and many can now be acquired while you are working, as well as through the traditional route of spending a year or more as a full-time college student.

The main body awarding qualifications in the social work field is the Central Council for Education and Training in Social Work (CCETSW). Its address is listed on page 162.

Qualifications

There is still plenty of interesting work that can be found by people without formal qualifications. Their 'qualifications' are their experience and their personality. But as you will probably already know, there may come a time when you realise that you are perfectly capable of doing better-paid and more demanding work, perhaps because your present job has brought you in contact with a district nurse, a social worker or some other professional colleague and you feel 'I could do that'. For most of these jobs you will need a qualification.

Qualifications can help you in all sorts of ways. Getting them will increase your confidence by broadening your base of knowledge and skills. Qualifications help employers because although they do not prove that you will be brilliant at a job, they tend to suggest that at least you are unlikely to fall below a minimum level. They also provide an impartial national standard which helps any employer weigh one candidate for a job against another. Increasingly, too, in a competitive world, qualified staff are considered a commercial asset – worth boasting about in a brochure. Indeed, in many situations, employers are legally obliged to employ staff who have a particular qualification or are on a statutory register – for instance, a nursing home must have Registered General Nurse on the staff.

Many people wanting to improve their qualifications start by thinking in terms of the traditional qualifications – GCSEs (which used to be called O levels), A levels and degrees. These may be the right ones for you, but you will already have seen from the preceding section that there are many, many more from which you can choose. For instance, City and Guilds offer a complete route to a professional career in care through their '325' certificates (see page 162); the Business Technician and Education Council (BTEC) awards management, business and technical qualifications; and the National Nursery Education Board (NNEB) oversees nursery nurses' qualifications.

When you are looking for a qualification that has 'cash value' in work terms, it might be wise to consider these less familiar qualifications. The traditional qualifications, such as GCSEs, tend to cater better for younger people than for adults, and specifically vocational qualifications may help you achieve your goal more quickly. Vocational qualifications will also, in the near future, all come under a new system called 'National Vocational Qualifications' which will put more emphasis on the practical skill you need for the job than academic knowledge and where the traditional memory-testing examination is replaced by more flexible, more practical and less terrifying methods of assessment.

Finding advice

Since the world of qualifications and training is a confusing and complicated scene, it is highly desirable to get advice on what will suit you. Reliable advice is patchily provided, but you might try any of these sources:

Local libraries

Libraries often contain a computer terminal with detailed practical advice, addresses, dates and times. Even where they do not, they normally carry pamphlets and brochures of all local organizations offering training. They also keep directories listing training, careers and qualifications. Among the titles to look out for are the following:

British Qualifications, 18th edition, Kogan Page, London (1988)
Segal, A., *Careers Encyclopaedia*, 12th edition, Cassell, London (1989)
Handbook of Free Careers Information in the UK, 4th edition, Careers Consultants, London (1987).

Training Access Points (TAPs)

These are computer terminals with local information on training. The idea is that they will eventually become available everywhere, but at the moment they are limited to a few libraries and job centres.

Educational Guidance Centres

These are sometimes run by local education authorities, often from slightly scruffy-looking lock-up shops which have become available on short leases. The advice is usually excellent and free.

Citizens Advice Bureaux (CABs)

CABs may sometimes be able to help, but their funding is under threat and as a result there may not be a branch near you or it may only be open at limited times.

Job centres

These should be able to advise on training as well as on current job vacancies.

Adult Education Centres
These can sometimes offer careers advice.

Writing direct to colleges and examining bodies

When you know roughly the subject area into which you want to
move, this is one of the most direct routes. Most examining bodies
publish helpful literature on careers and qualifications, including lists
of colleges offering individual courses. Here are some useful addresses:

National Board for Nursing, Midwifery and Health Visiting for
Scotland
22 Queen Street
Edinburgh EH2 1JX

Welsh National Board for Nursing, Midwifery and Health Visiting
Pearl Assurance House
Greyfriars Road
Cardiff CF1 3AG

English National Board for Nursing, Midwifery and Health Visiting
Victory House
170 Tottenham Court Road
London W1P 0AH

National Board for Nursing, Midwifery and Health Visiting for
Northern Ireland
RAC House
Chichester Street
Belfast BT1 4JE

Central Council for Education and Training in Social Work
Information Service
Derbyshire Houses
St Chad's Street
London WC1H 8AD

City and Guilds of London Institute
46 Britannia Street
London WC1X 9RG

National Council for Vocational Qualifications
222 Euston Road
London NW1 2BZ

Business and Technician Educational Council (BTEC)
Tavistock House
Tavistock Square
London WC1H 9LG

Choosing a training course

Training courses vary greatly in their quality. Probably most people have had experiences like this:

> I went on a course about means-tested grants. It lasted a day and consisted of one person after another standing up and lecturing us. I felt completely bamboozled at the end of it. I wondered later why they hadn't just sent us the handouts and not bothered with the expense of the trip to London.

> I didn't learn anything – I felt everyone there probably knew more than me and I never got over my nerves. It was just one boring lecture after another. There was a bit of discussion but I felt too timid to join in.

This kind of training is very unlikely to be effective. The fact that you are not involved means that your attention is likely to wander: adults can only concentrate on information that is given verbally for about ten minutes at the most. This kind of method also means that the teacher or trainer is only getting very limited feedback from the group so cannot adjust his or her performance accordingly: it may be too difficult for some of the group and too easy for others, but a trainer who teaches using these methods is unlikely to find out which.

Most adults feel nervous at the beginning of a course: worrying, for instance, about the possibility of looking silly in front of other people, or about whether they will be able to keep up with the work. A good trainer will find ways of helping people on the course overcome these nerves by reassuring them, making the first tasks simple ones, creating opportunities for members of the group to get to know each other, and sharing the purpose of the course by making its objectives crystal clear.

The effective trainer also designs the learning around *doing* rather than listening or watching. There's no getting away from the truth of that old Chinese proverb which says: 'I hear and I forget. I see and I remember. I do and I understand.' Imagine you are going to learn how to do a particular kind of lift. You have three options: to hear someone describe it; to see someone do it; and to do it yourself with someone to guide you. A verbal description and a demonstration would no doubt be helpful, but it is unlikely that you would learn quickly or effectively by listening and watching. The only real way to learn how to lift is to *do* it.

So good trainers will make every minute count by building in plenty of practical activity and plenty of participation from the group: role-plays where two or more people 'act out' a difficult situation which is then discussed by the group, discussions, projects and so on, with a minimum of lecturing from the trainer. These methods also draw on the lecturers' own experience: the only sensible way to proceed with adults who often have a lot to contribute, as this social work trainer comments:

> I teach young graduates and mature people on day release who often have many years of practical experience behind them. The graduates are confident and sparky, but the real pleasure is teaching the mature learners. They just won't let you get away with anything. If they don't find a particular theory convincing they say so because they know from the field how much theory differs from practice. I have learnt so much from them!

Feedback has already been mentioned in this chapter because of its importance in relation to your normal work. It is equally important on a training course. Not being given feedback can be maddening, as this learner comments:

> I did a nursery nursing course but I found it extremely frustrating. Our essays and practicals were marked but we never knew why we'd got the marks we had. If you got a low mark you felt terribly cast down because you never knew why, or what to do to put it right. But equally, if you got a high mark it could leave you baffled, too, because you didn't know why it was good, so you weren't sure how to get it again.

On the other hand, being given detailed feedback in the right way can have a startlingly positive effect. Here is the other side of the story:

> We had a tremendously good tutor on a short course I did. We had to do a project on one client. The tutor helped us plan every stage of it and because she gave us such detailed comment on the outline, we were very much less likely to go wrong later, but also her comments on the submitted projects were great.

She showed she understood what you were trying to say and gave you terrific ideas on where to improve. It inspired me so much that I went on to do the qualification.

Summing up then, this checklist will help you judge the quality of the teaching on a training course. Ticks in every column indicate a high-calibre course

The trainer makes the aims and objectives clear ☐

There is a minimum of lecturing and being 'talked at' ☐

Active methods of learning are used such as
discussion, practice, role-play ☐

Learners are constantly asked for their experience ☐

Learners get consistent and helpful feedback on their
work ☐

Open learning

For many people, a full-time training course is out of the question. Their domestic commitments are too heavy, or they simply cannot afford to stop earning while they are learning (even though for work-related courses, as we have seen, the employer may pay the fees). Open learning is an attractive alternative to the traditional course in such cases. With an open learning course, the lectures and discussions of traditional teaching are replaced by a 'package' – typically workbooks that you write in, perhaps a course textbook, a video and some audiotapes. You submit assignments to a tutor and may have to complete some practical assessments as well. The Open University provides degree courses in a wide range of subjects and also offers a course for care workers called *Caring for Older People* (course P650). Information is available from:

Student Enquiry Service
The Open University
Walton Hall
Milton Keynes
MK7 6AA

The Open College also has a popular course specifically for care support workers. It is called *The Carers* and can lead to the City and

Guilds certificate in Community Care Practice (325). To find out more, write to:

The Open College
St James's Buildings
Oxford Street
Manchester
M1 6FO

Summary

This chapter has briefly described some of the possibilities for moving on, starting from consolidating the skills in the job done currently and moving on into care management, nursing and allied fields or social work. The importance of improving qualifications is emphasized together with some advice on how to judge the calibre of the teaching on a course and where to find educational advice and guidance.

Booklist

This short booklist contains some suggestions for further reading. They are included either because they are classics on the subject, or because of their pithiness and practicality.

Dickson, A. (1982) *A Woman in Your Right*, Quartet Books, London. One of the best introductions to assertiveness, what it means and how to put it into practice.

First Aid Manual (1987) fifth edition, Dorling Kindersley, London. The classic first-aid reference book: brief, very well illustrated and not expensive to buy. It is endorsed by all three British first-aid organizations.

Goffman, E. (1968), *Asylums*, Penguin, Harmondsworth. The classic study of the effects of institutions on people. This book has been influential in raising uncomfortable questions about the purposes and value of institutional care.

Kubler-Ross, E. (1982) *Living with Death and Dying*, Souvenir Press, London.

Murray–Parkes, C. (1986) *Bereavement: Studies of Grief in Adult Life*, Revised edition, Penguin, Harmondsworth. A dense but readable account of the effects of loss.

Newton, E. (1980) *This Bed My Centre*, Virago, London. A vivid personal account of what it feels like to be a client.

Norman, A. (1987), *Aspects of Ageism*, Centre for Policy on Ageing, London. A challenging, thought provoking book on how prejudice contaminates dealings with old people.

Norman, A. (1987) *Rights and Risk*, Centre for Policy on Ageing, London.
A challenging and readable short book with a full discussion on issues relating to assessing risks in caring for clients.

Office of the Minister for the Civil Service (1987) *Understanding Stress*, HMSO, London.

Reader's Digest Association (1986) *What To Do in an Emergency*.
An excellent reference book with ideas on preventing and dealing with a wide range of emergencies, including fire.

Stokes, G. (1987) *Incontinence and Inappropriate Urinating*, Winslow Press, Bicester.
One of several brief, practical books by the same author on dealing with the management of confused clients.

Townsend, P. (1963) *The Family Life of Old People*, Penguin, Harmondsworth.
Readable and racy account, based on the author's research in the East End of London.

Index